FOLK AND FESTIVAL
Costume

FOLK AND FESTIVAL
Costume

A Historical Survey with Over 600 Illustrations

R. TURNER WILCOX

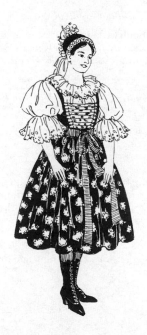

DOVER PUBLICATIONS, INC.
Mineola, New York

Bibliographical Note

This Dover edition, first published in 2011, is an unabridged republication of the work originally published by Charles Scribner's Sons, New York, in 1965 under the title *Folk and Festival Costume of the World.*

Library of Congress Cataloging-in-Publication Data

Wilcox, R.Turner (Ruth Turner), 1888–1970.
   [Folk and festival costume of the world]
   Folk and festival costume : a historical survey with over 600 illustrations / R. Turner Wilcox.
      p. cm.
   "This Dover edition, first published in 2011, is an unabridged republication of the work originally published by Charles Scribner's Sons, New York, in 1965 under the title Folk and Festival Costume of the World."
   Includes bibliographical references and index.
   ISBN-13: 978-0-486-47871-5
   ISBN-10: 0-486-47871-8
   1. Clothing and dress—History. 2. Clothing and dress—History—Pictorial works. I. Title.

GT510.W54 2011
391.009—dc22

2010040189

Manufactured in the United States by Courier Corporation
47871801
www.doverpublications.com

to Ray Wilcox and Ruth Wilcox

❧ Contents ❧

❈ *Foreword* ❈

The wearing of folk costume is on the decline in many countries and this is an effort to record, before too late, what remains of so charming a custom. A feeling of sentiment for the old and an appreciation of the artistic has prompted some educators to revise the usage and persuade some of their provincial groups not to discard regional costume.

The dress of the peasant has of necessity always differed from that worn by his betters because of his work and the need of strong fiber in his clothes to withstand hard wear. And even were he able to afford good cloth, he was prohibited from wearing it by sumptuary decrees which not only banned the use of fine fabric but the use of beautiful color as well. Too, he was limited in dyes and compelled to use earth colors which furnished the prevalent gray, brown and dull green. Of simplest design and fashioned of coarse homespun, dress proclaimed the peasant's status in society.

Sumptuary laws against extravagant raiment date back to Bible times, were common in ancient Greece and Rome and so strictly enforced in the 14th and 15th centuries in Europe that penalties in fines were imposed upon those who disobeyed. This was the case even in the American Colonies at a later date.

The 16th century witnessed the passing of the Medieval feudal order along with its moralists and reformers. Part of the religious zeal of these latter was directed against the extreme Italian fashions of the period, demanding instead neutral colors, plain cloth and a specific form of dress for each class, nobility, the middle class and the peasantry. It was contended that an individual's class should be apparent in his dress.

The settling of the new continents in the 16th and 17th centuries of the Renaissance period and the ensuing increase in commerce and wealth which was confined not only to the nobility but the upper class, gave rise to ostentatious display in dress. Handsome Oriental fabrics such as brocades, velvets, gold lace, feathers, jewels and an apparently inexhaustible supply of fine furs from the New World became available to the bourgeoisie.

Though the Church had long worn gorgeous robes, it disapproved of the extravagance of the nobles but did not dare rebuke the wearers. Instead, the rich clothes of the rising wealthy merchants were noted and disapproval shown by the passing of more sumptuary laws. The peasants who were equally desirous of festive Sunday garments took to ornamenting their homespun with colorful hand stitchery and beautiful handmade lace. The simple white linen chemise, shirte (sic) or smock naively and artistically enriched and worn with dark cloth masculine breeches or feminine skirt became the costume for Church and gala occasions.

As the years passed and the embroidery became more and more elaborate, the pieces were kept in handsome wooden chests and handed on as precious heirlooms, being worn from generation to generation. Men became as skillful embroiderers as the women, with whole families spending the long winter evenings, when fieldwork was impossible, in designing and stitching colorful motifs on their garments.

Except perhaps in some detail of embroidery or lace, there was no change in style. The bride-to-be spent her early years in preparing her wedding trousseau and linen and if her parents were wealthy, she would carry many well-filled chests to her new home. Invariably, the handsomely embroidered wedding chemise of the groom had been the loving handwork of the girl.

In the 17th century the elegant Spanish fashions which long had exercised an influence upon the mode of European courts became familiar enough to the peasantry for them to incorporate some of the ideas into their own dress. Such were the masculine doublet or short jacket and the laced feminine corseted bodice, both of which have remained important features of folk dress to our day.

A study of regional dress reveals the tendency towards creating a national look which can be noted especially in Italian, German and Protestant Central Europe. Unique design was the result of living in a village hemmed in by mountains and far from a travelled road. Costumes were not always uniform in style and color, the maker and wearer often adding a bit of her own creativeness to the work. In general, however, there was enough similarity in the dress of a given village to tell an outsider the wearer's home and social status. One notes that the maiden was distinguishable from the matron and that a Protestant would be known from a Catholic.

For instance, in England there appeared the Puritan garb of the Cromwellian Period, 1649 to 1660. Of course, the Puritans did not create a style but simply denuded the mode of its fripperies, resulting in an outer covering that "told all" about the wearer.

A fashion in those days lasted a century or more and peasant dress did not become "folk dress" until around 1800 when it developed into festival dress for Church, weddings, christenings and funerals. For the latter use, the addition of a mourning badge on sleeve or headgear was sufficient, such as the black crêpe sleeve-band which was worn on a man's tweed suit in the 19th century.

Such is the story of folk dress in the western world but there is also the story of Eastern, Oriental and African dress, of beautifully woven lengths of cloth draped round the body in picturesque folds. Still the national dress of various countries with temperate weather, it is simple and artistic but impractical. Of cloth of grass, cotton, linen and wool, it is usually a handwoven, straight length of uncut fabric that must be arranged about the figure with each wearing. In this style of costume the ancient Greeks and Romans perfected the art of drapery for all time.

Though regional dress is worn in many lands, modern machinery is slowly pushing it to one side. In this 20th century the world is becoming politically, commercially and socially quite closely knit, with people adopting better ways of doing things from each other. Machine-made cloth is more durable and at the same time makes a better garb for working in the field. More suitable to farming, or in general for factory work, are the western machine-sewn denim jacket, breeches and overalls. But, as one sighs again, efficiency dispenses with artistry.

FOLK AND FESTIVAL
Costume

❈ *Afghanistan* ❈

Plate 1

Afghanistan is today a country of Central Asia lying between Iran, the Soviet Union and India. Its people have a diverse ethnic background but they have a point of unity in their Islamic religion and culture. As Moslems, the women lead secluded harem lives, most women still going completely shrouded when in public. Desert-dwelling wives were permitted by the Koran to go unveiled.

1. Afghan tribesman in general dress except for leather belts and arms. Full, wrapped pantaloons or "tombons" and loose tunic of white cotton. Waistcoat of red felt or sheepskin. Low leather shoes with turned-up toes. Turban of white cotton, a straight piece of cloth 20 to 30 inches wide and 6 to 9 yards in length. As a Moslem, the turban is so draped that the forehead is bare to touch the ground when the wearer prays to Allah. In winter, he adds a greatcoat of sheepskin, felt or woolen cloth.

2. Red waistcoat of felt, cloth or dyed sheepskin heavily embroidered with gold braid.

3. Pillbox of black velvet and bright colored silk with heavy gold embroidery worn under the enveloping chadar, a coverall wrap. Married women wear their hair plaited or dressed up under the cap while that of unmarried girls hangs flowing or in ringlets.

4. Upper class woman in street dress wearing the chadar which she would hold together up to her eyes. This concealing garb is worn in gray, beige, light or dark blue cotton, silk or calico. Under it, the full, draped tombons and tunic which might be of cotton or silk and the short, sleeveless jacket of velvet, silk or cotton with embroidery.

5. Upper class man in white tombons, pleated tunic with embroidered bodice and sleeves. Embroidered cloth waistcoat. All embroidery in dark red silk spangled with tiny mirrors. Turban of red and white silk, and peaked-toe leather shoes of Turkish style.

6. Young prince in white muslin tombons and tunic. Embroidery in red, over-stitched with yellow, green and black accents. Folded, sleeveless jacket over arm in black cloth with red and gold embroidery. Also over arm, a loongee, folded handkerchief of cotton or silk used for sash or over shoulder. Low leather shoes, bone color with red.

7. Black waistcoat of felt, cloth or dyed sheepskin heavily embroidered with silver braid.

8. A farmer in white cotton tombons and tunic. Tunic skirt held up by the loongee cloth tied around waist. Tail of turban over shoulder serves as dust veil, purse, pocket handkerchief or whatever.

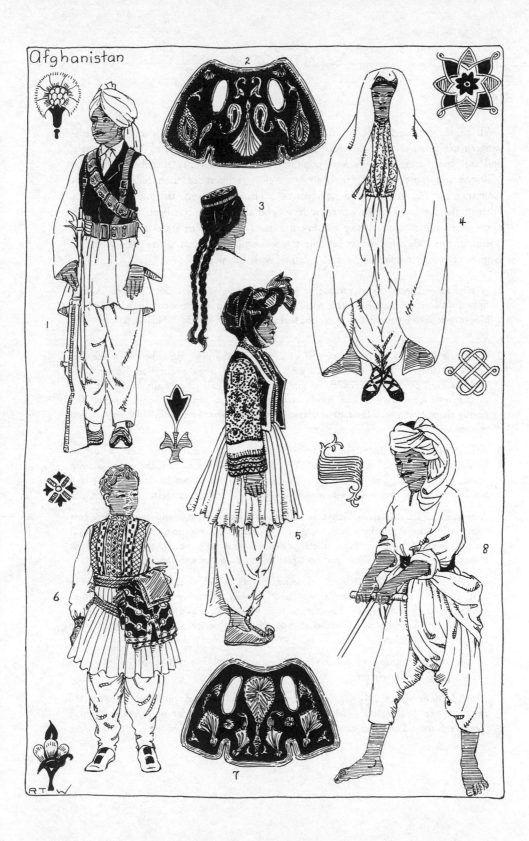

Afghanistan

❧ *Africa* ❧

Plate 2

Africa, the second largest continent in the eastern hemisphere, forms the south-western extension of Asia to which it is attached by the Isthmus of Suez. Climate and soil have caused the various populations to be unevenly distributed. Native religions and the power of fetishism are followed by more than half of the inhabitants, the remainder being devotees of Mohammedanism, the most important faith of the continent. A beneficent effect upon the natives has been that of Islam upon heathendom. Christianity has taken a hold, a Christian state being Ethiopia. Africa of the 20th century has become the scene of nationalist aspirations with the Negroes of today demanding racial equality with the whites.

1. A woman of Liberia in a costume of many colors. A sash-tied skirt printed in red, brown and yellow and bordered with black silk. With it she wears a white cotton blouse printed in pale colors. Her tied-turban is also of cotton in black striped with pink.

2. A unique headdress worn by women of a tribe of the Nyangara region in the Republic of Congo. The skulls of both men and women from infancy are drawn back and distorted by means of bands of giraffe hide and hair, the bands being replaced as the head grows larger. The bands in the illustration appear to be fine wire. The flaring shape over which the hair is dressed is either of wire or wood. Worn by married women.

3. A man of Dakar of the Republic of Senegal is shown wearing the kibr, a sort of tight-fitting gaberdine in striped silk or cotton. It is worn over the tobe, a long white cotton shirt. The kibr pictured is slit up to the knees in front and has a hood in back. He wears a multicolored skullcap and leather sandals.

4. A woman of the Masai in Kenya is coiffed with shaved head and wire fillets. Her costume of brown goatskins is not unlike a modern Paris creation. All her "jewelry," anklets, armlets, necklaces and fillets, some threaded with beads, are of copper or iron wire and her ears are slashed, not pierced, to hold her earrings.

5. A college man of Ibadan, Nigeria, wearing the aba which does service as coat, over-coat, raincoat or blanket. Usually woven of camel's hair or wool in black, orange, brown or cream-color but in this case, of thin white cotton and breeches of the same, for summer. A white cotton tarboosh-type cap and leather shoes of Western style complete the costume.

6. A woman of Monrovia in Liberia in a handsome self-tied turban of heavy cotton striped pink and raspberry.

7. Also of Monrovia in Liberia, this youngster wears a cotton tunic edged with red cotton fringe. It is striped with red and orange, the red circles on a white ground. The wrap-around undergarment is of white cotton.

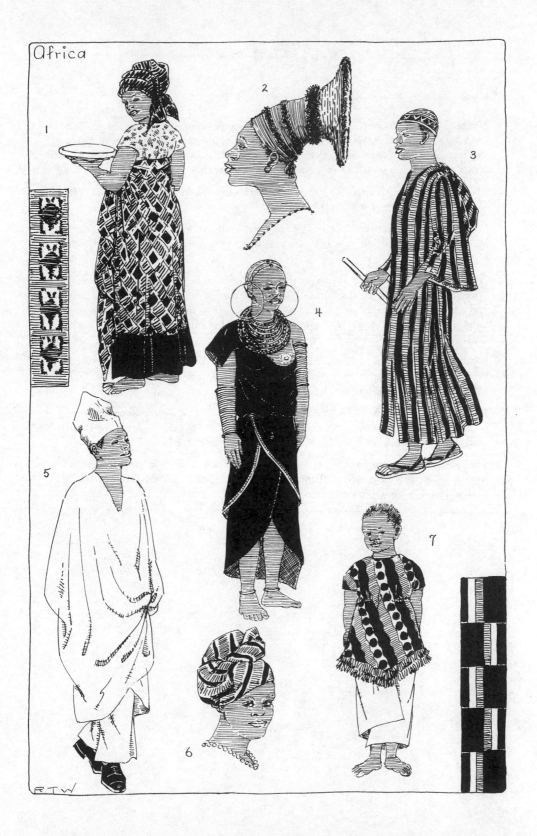

❋ *Africa* ❋

Plate 3

1. Native of Lorian Swamp, Kenya, a Mohammedan sheik in a striking aba. White cloth with wide border, probably red with a single yellow stripe. Under it, he wears the tobe, a white cotton shirt reaching to the ankles; an unusually-draped white cotton turban, white socks and Western style leather shoes.

2. The Mohammedan trader of Monrovia in Liberia wears a knitted white cotton cap with wide stripes of brown and black.

3. College man of Ibadan in Nigeria wearing the white cotton aba over dark cloth Western breeches and leather shoes. His cap of variegated colors is either knitted or embroidered.

4. A flower-seller of Durban's Indian quarter in South Africa. His smock-like robe is a long white cotton shirt, the kŭrtă. It has a red border, is fastened at the left side and the long shirt sleeves are fastened at the wrist. His turban or pagri is of cotton in alternating stripes in red and white or cream color. Attached to his belt are a red and white fabric envelope purse and a watch.

5. A woman of Monrovia, Liberia, wearing an arresting, colorful cotton print in red, black and white. The wrap-around skirt is tied and tucked in at the waist in front. Her smart made-up turban is white cotton striped with gray and black.

6. A young Wagogo man of Tanganyika wears his hair long while the young women crop theirs closely. The tiny pigtails are plastered with red ochre which, combined with the dark skin, gives a wig-like effect. Slashed ears hold the beaded wire earrings.

7. The lace and ribbon-trimmed lingerie dress of white lawn is worn by an East Indian woman of Natal, South Africa. Tunic and skirt are further embellished with pink ribbon. Her headscarf is sheer white.

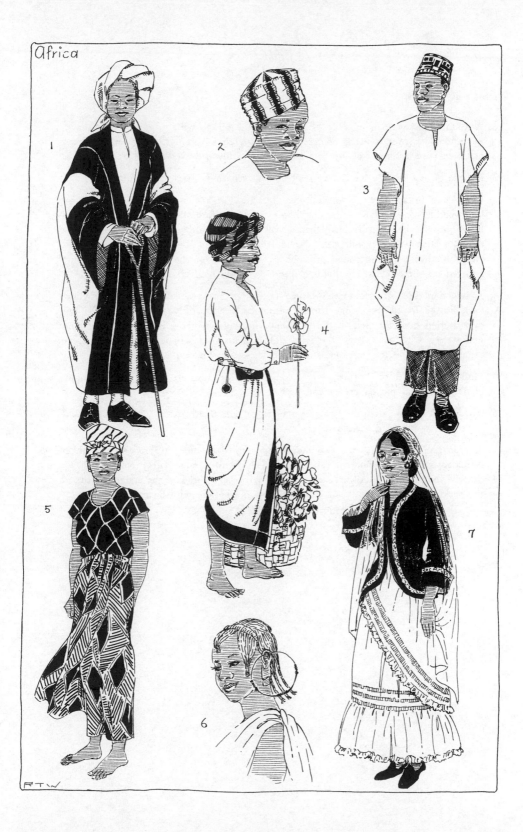

Africa

❈ *Africa* ❈

Plate 4

1. A young Zulu woman of Port Elizabeth, South Africa, with a draped silk shawl, red and black over a black bodice. Anklets, bracelets, earrings, necklace and head ornaments are fashioned of tiny, white porcelain beadwork, even to her walking stick.

2. A little girl's headdress of closely plaited hair seen in Nigeria and Ethiopia.

3. A Ndebele bride of the Transvaal, South Africa, in a remarkable cloak worn on her wedding day and never again. Three months before the event, a sheepskin is fashioned and her friends busy themselves with the handwork. In our illustration the skin is shown black, all else of solid white beading. The neckrings and anklets are of beadwork wound round grass hoops, dark blue for the neck and blue, white and red for the anklets. She holds a wedding stick which is also beaded.

4. A Nigerian chief dressed for a Moslem festival in a superb aba of cloth in white, dark blue and red. His huge turban, also red, is beautifully draped with the tail over the left shoulder as it should be. Kano, northern Nigeria, is famous for dyeing white cloth with color from the wild indigo plant into wonderful shades of blue ranging from pale to deep tones, the latter especially favored by the Tuaregs.

5. Mother and child of Yoruba, Nigeria. Baby is traveling in a "picken." Turban, blouse, skirt and picken are of cotton.

6. An infant of the Ndebele Tribe in the Transvaal, South Africa, with the tiniest curls ever. White bead neck-hoop.

7. A Ndebele woman in a smart winter wrap. The dark blue and red wool blanket is folded over into a shoulder cape and fastened with a huge safety pin. The head-dress is composed of beadwork and coins. Also of beadwork are the square motifs of the necklace. The wire anklets are finished top and bottom with bead hoops.

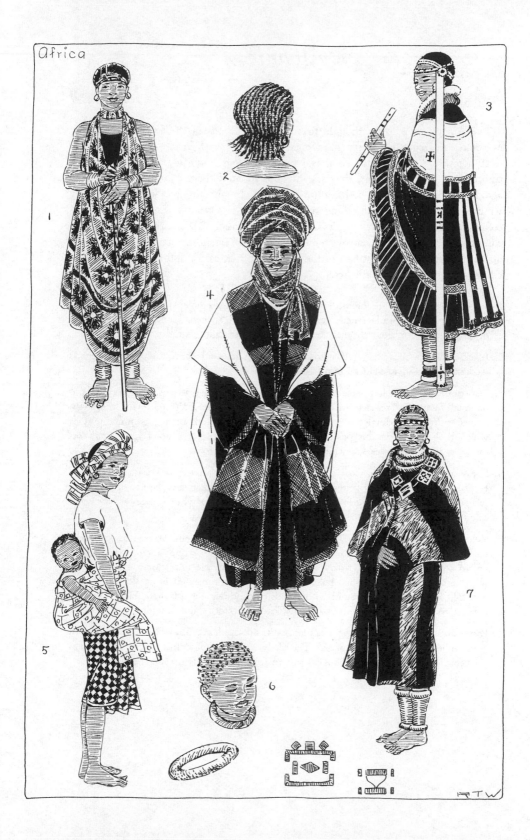

Africa

❧ *Albania* ❧

Plate 5   see TURKEY

The Albanians, who are thought to be the descendants of the earliest Aryan immigrants, are regarded as the most ancient race of southeastern Europe. History does not record their origin or arrival in the Balkan Peninsula. A turbulent, untutored but virtuous people, they fought hard to hold their mountain strongholds against the many odds of both nature and man. Finally in the 15th century, they were overcome by the Turks and made part of the Ottoman Empire, which accounts for the Turkish style of dress and ornamentation. Today, they are a Balkan communist republic in a narrow mountainous land extending along the east coast of the Adriatic. The largest part of the population is Moslem, followed by Orthodox Christians and Roman Catholics.

1. White linen chemise or blouse and skirt. White woolen bolero embroidered in gay colors. Apron of hand-loomed woolen cloth, Roman striped. Cummerbund of wool or heavy silk. Embroidered headkerchief worn over calotte or cap.

2. Black velvet tarboosh covered with gold fringe and gold coins, the coins given as wedding gifts, an age-old custom.

3. Fur-trimmed black cloth bolero called a Scanderberg after the Albanian chief and national hero who resisted the Turks from 1443 to 1468. White linen shirt with striped cuffs. Full pantaloons or chalwar held by wide cloth or silk cummerbund in which the man carries his possessions, money, pipe, tobacco, a good knife and, formerly, a pistol. He wears a white felt tarboosh.

4. Dress for gala occasions. Coat of dark colored cloth or velvet, stiff with heavy gold embroidery, braid and paillettes. Sheer white blouse of linen and lace. Cummerbund securing the dark green satin chalwar. Headcloth of crisp white gauze worn over a calotte. Embroidered peak-toed slippers of Turkish style.

5. Gentleman's dress for official and gala functions. The fustanella or pleated kilt, relic of ancient Greek and Roman times. Tunic and kilt of white linen. Black velvet bolero solidly embroidered with gold braid. Simulated effect of three jackets which was the original form. Slashed bolero sleeves permit the pleated tunic sleeves to flare out. Silk or velvet cummerbund with exquisite handkerchief attached. Heavy knitted hose worn like boots and gartered. Black leather Oxfords and a white felt tarboosh.

6. Party dress with chalwar of polka dot pink silk foulard. Black velvet bolero with gold embroidery. Turban of gauze. The chalwar, either masculine or feminine, takes a piece of fabric measuring about 90 square feet or 10 yards of 36″ material.

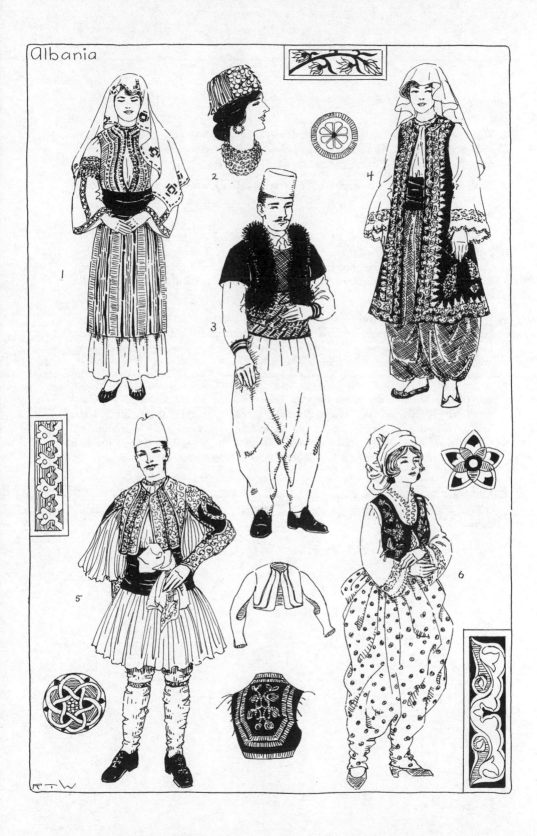

Albania

❧ *Albania* ❧

Plate 6

1. White chiffon blouse with chalwar of delicate peach-colored satin brocade. Fringed sash of taffeta checked in black and white. Black velvet bolero ornamented with rows of gold fringe. Pleated gauze headscarf. (1930's)

2. Small boy in heavy white cotton or linen with colored woolen waistcoat and cummerbund of striped silk. White felt calotte or skullcap and leather shoes with turned-up toes.

3. A rich outfit in plum color. Cloth coat with plum-colored braid embroidery. The cuffs, fringed sash and side panel of the chalwar are of scarlet moiré silk. White chiffon blouse or chemise shows above and below a solidly gold-embroidered deep-cut bolero. Headkerchief of embroidered white gauze secured by a jeweled fillet. Gold embroidered mules.

4. White cloth breeches with low-cut crotch and low-hung pouch pockets. Striped fabric cummerbund sashed with red silk. Violet cloth bolero buttoned-trimmed. Embroidered white waistcoat. The modern collar signifies a modern Western shirt. White felt tarboosh and black leather shoes.

5. A bride in her wedding finery. White linen skirt and blouse with flaring, pleated sleeves. The omnipresent homespun woolen apron in Roman-striped coloring. Sumptuous fringed silk sash tied round the waist in cummerbund fashion. Black velvet bolero covered with gold coins handed down from generation to generation for bridal wear. Around her neck hang beads, chains and several crucifixes. Bracelets on her arms and rings on all her fingers. Hair and eyebrows dyed black and her fingers henna'd.

6. Little girl in white cotton chemise with the usual bolero and apron, both of bright colored woolen cloth. Underneath, the white chalwar and leather shoes with turned-up toes.

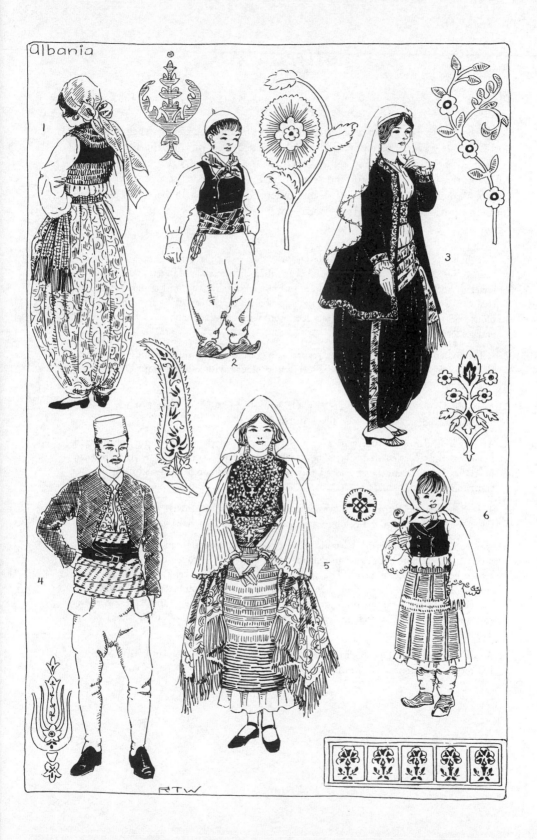

Albania

❊ Algeria ❊

Plate 7   see BARBARY STATES, BEDOUINS

Algeria forms part of the southern shore of the Mediterranean between Morocco and Libya. It was conquered by the Vandals in the 5th century, by the East Roman Empire in the 6th century and by the Arabs in the 7th century. From 1705, it was ruled by the Ottoman Empire and from 1830 by the French. It was politically a part of France until 1962 when it became independent. Arabs, Berbers, and Kabyles form the predominant race groups today and Roman Catholicism is the chief religion.

1. The haik, a long piece of white cotton or woolen cloth according to weather, envelops the Algerian woman in public. In this picture, a gold belt clasped by a jeweled buckle holds it in blouse-like fashion. A "fall" veil hides her face. The chalwar is a deep sky-blue satin brocade probably topped by a loose, over-hanging blouse of sheer white fabric. On her feet, soft white leather babouches worked with embroidery.

2. A barefooted little girl in a red fez secured decoratively by a multicolored silk square. With it she wears an embroidered sheer white blouse with lace edging. The chalwar is of bright pink figured cotton.

3. A lovely bonnet for special occasions. Of gauze embroidered in soft tones of blue and rose, accented with gold or silver stitchery.

4. An Algerian dancer in full, scarlet satin chalwar with black velvet bolero embroidered in silver and ivory-colored silk. The black velvet cap is decorated with a brooch, pearl beads and some ivory-colored tail feathers. Rose-colored suède slippers are accompanied by gold anklets.

5. The Caid or tribal magistrate wears a vermilion cloth burnous with white hood. Over the hood, a large varicolored straw hat which lends a halo look to the wearer.

6. and 7. The circular-shaped burnous with hood woven in one piece is usually put on over the turban although this falconer wears his turban over the hood. There is also a burnous without hood. The gandoura, an African sleeveless robe, is of white cotton or wool. The illustration shows the Western man's cloth jacket and white cotton shirt which have been quite generally adopted in the cities. Our Algerian wears soft shoes with socks which many men keep on when taking off their shoes before entering the Mosque.

8. A little girl in pale blue bodice, chalwar of printed violet cotton and, tied over her red fez, a rose-colored silk headkerchief.

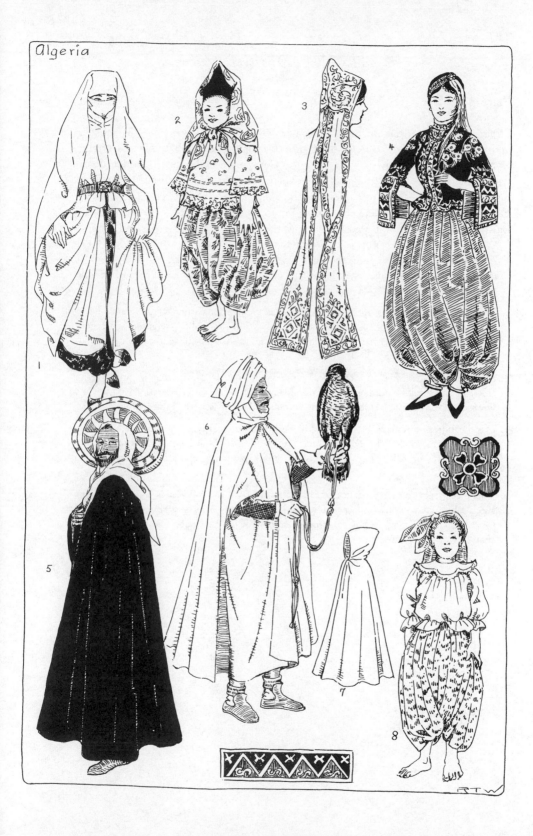

Algeria

❧ *Alsace-Lorraine* ❧

Plate 8   see FRANCE

Alsace-Lorraine forms a frontier region between France, Germany, Luxembourg and Switzerland. At the close of the Franco-Prussian War in 1871, Alsace-Lorraine along with several subdivisions was ceded to Germany. While under German domination all attempts to Germanize the country were strongly resisted. Particularly disturbing was the religious question, the greater part of the population being Catholic. The provinces were restored to France by the treaty of Versailles in 1919. Bas-Rhin, Haut-Rhin and Moselle are now the French names for Alsace-Lorraine.

1. A doll-like little lady wearing the huge black taffeta bowknot and the black corselet laced with black ribbons. The blouse and apron are of white lawn and white lisle stockings and black slippers complete the costume.

2. The traditional dress of an Alsatian mayor and chief magistrate of a village. Navy blue serge cloth with the tricolor sash of red, white and blue weighted with gold tassels. During the German occupation, only the sash was changed to the German colors of red, white and black.

3. A frilled, lace-trimmed cap of sheer white lawn that folds up like a fan. Over a frock of gold color cashmere is worn a black silk apron embroidered in pink. The wrap is a fringed shawl of dark blue woven with stripes of a lighter blue.

4. Her headdress of heavy bright red silk designates the lady as a Catholic. She also favors plaid silks for the bowknot. Her skirt is red with a bolero blouse of dark colored velvet or silk. The apron of sheer white lawn is elaborately embroidered in white.

5. The black silk bowknot of heavy silk tells one that the wearer is Protestant. The sheer white lawn blouse is lace-trimmed and accompanied by a dark green silk skirt. Over the latter, a black silk apron embroidered with blue flowers. The knotted fringed shawl is of changeable silk.

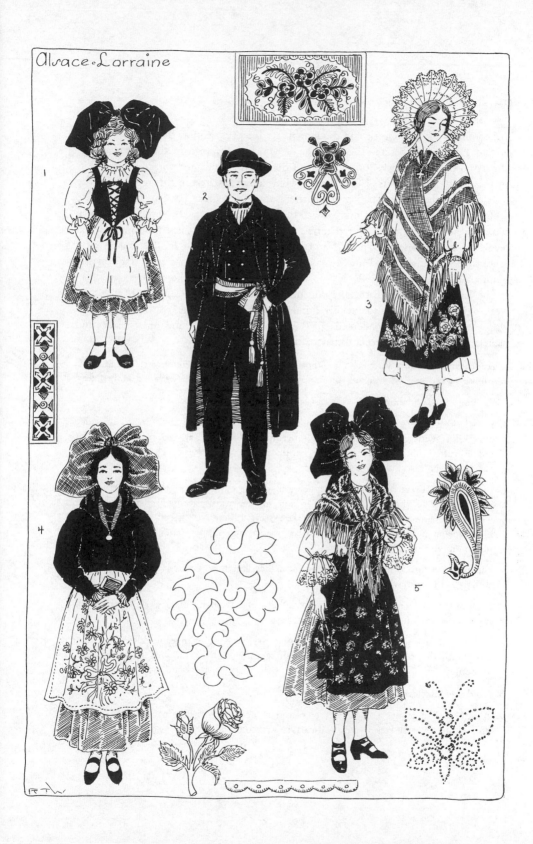

Alsace-Lorraine

❊ *Anatolia* ❊

Plate 9   see TURKEY

Anatolia is the late Greek and modern name for Asia Minor, the western peninsula of Asia which became the Ottoman or Turkish Empire in the 13th century. On its north is the Black Sea, the Aegean Sea on the west, and the Mediterranean on the south. Three fifths of the Turkish vilayets are situated in this region. By the 16th century the Empire had overrun the East and a great part of Europe. The decline in the next several centuries was due to exhausting wars, revolts of captive countries and loss of captured territories. In 1908 the young Turk movement led a revolt for reform and in World War I Turkey became one of the Central Powers of Europe. The first president, Mustafa Kemal Atatürk, set up a new state on the Plain of Anatolia and in 1923, he proclaimed Turkey a republic.

The Latin alphabet replaced the difficult Arabic script. In 1928, church and state were separated. Islam as the state religion was abolished. The wearing of the fez was abolished and men adopted the tailored Western costume of trousers and jacket. And women were permitted to unveil the face.

1. A peasant spinning yarn with a whorl. Chalwar of heavy cotton in French blue. Blouse of red and white plaid cotton. White headcloth bordered with red embroidery.

2. A "lion" in solid embroidery.

3. Bridal dress—chalwar and entari or tunic of delicately figured silk. Bolero in faded blue velvet with gold embroidery. Cummerbund of orange and red striped silk. The fez in tufted silk with a crown-like band of red velvet. Peak-toed shoes in either red velvet or soft kid.

4. Bridegroom's dress rich with embroidery, black on dark blue cloth. Simulated three waistcoats. The chalwar and lower section of the waistcoat of French blue cloth. The wide cummerbund is a Tunisian silk scarf in orange striped with red. Dark blue woolen hose and white gaiters. Red garters, red slippers and a red fez with a luxuriant blue silk tassel.

5. Peasant in a tarboosh covered with a cotton headkerchief, printed black on red. Red cotton band with white flower design.

6. Embroidery motif in gold and red from the back of a woman's black cloth bolero reaching from below the neckline to the waist.

7. A homemade cap of white felt with a puggree band of changeable black and blue silk. Until this century, all clothes for both sexes, except for the wealthy, were made at home.

8. Gold and silk brocading on linen.

9. A little girl in blouse and chalwar of cotton in deep, bright blue patterned with pink and white flowers. Her white headscarf is striped in pink.

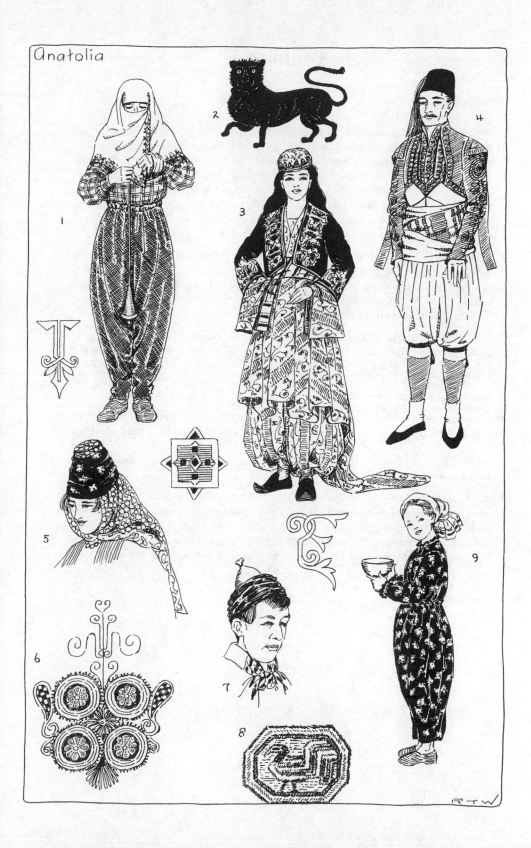

Anatolia

❧ *Anatolia* ❧

Plate 10

1. A Kurdish woman wearing what is considered a practical dress for performing her many and various chores, among them tending cattle. Under the entari or shift sashed with a self-cummerbund she wears a chalwar of striped cotton which is tucked into the peak-toed shoes. These latter are of red morocco leather. By way of repetition, the cummerbund serves not only the purpose of stomach band but as the carryall for what a Western woman carries in her handbag. The bolero is in a lovely faded blue color with gold embroidery. Her draped "fez" is red with blue silk tassel and draped round with a large flowered cotton handkerchief.

2. A bourgeois or business man of Manissa. He wears the white cotton shirt and with it a waistcoat and chalwar of red cloth. The costume is enriched by a cummerbund of white silk embroidered with small flowers in light colors. A fine color note is the bolero in soft, dark green cloth. His fez is red with the blue tassel and he wears white socks with black leather shoes.

3. A Moslem peasant in a simple costume which is richly enhanced by silver and gold coins suspended by fine chains attached to the tarboosh and the necklace. Chemise and bolero are of pink and white striped silk and the chalwar of Chinese blue cloth. The Tunisian cummerbund is of orange and yellow silk. White socks and red babouches complete the attire.

4. An artisan of Angora wearing her hair over her right shoulder in "pony tail" fashion. Her red fez has a silver embroidered crown, gold tassel, and is draped with a white muslin handkerchief painted with tiny flowers. Bolero and chalwar are of white silk striped and flowered, and, over the chalwar, a red and white striped cotton caftan. Her babouches are yellow morocco.

5. An Israelite professor in town costume from Smyrna. His white turban, called a bonneto, is unlike the broad Moslem style. His chalwar is of gray cotton, the caftan of blue and white striped silk and the voluminous cloak of red cloth. Round his waist, a gray cashmere sash striped and fringed in red. With red morocco leather babouches he wears yellow socks and carries a handsome cane of cherry-wood.

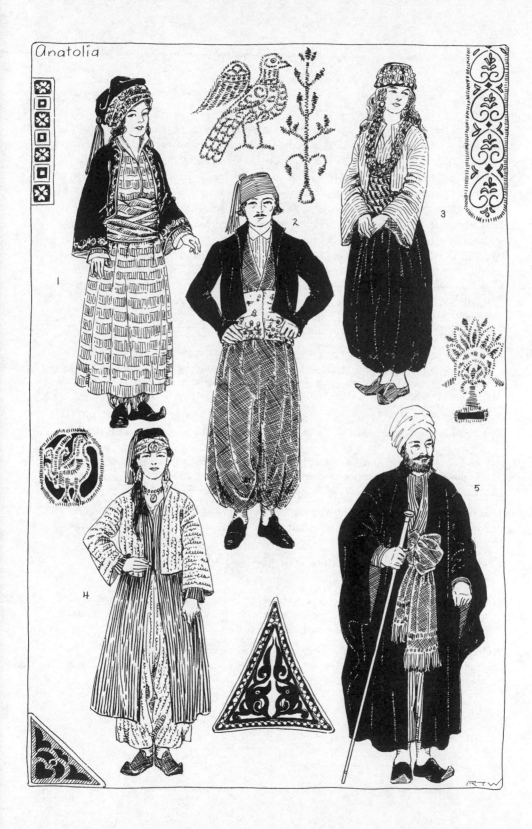

Anatolia

❊ *Arabia* ❊

Plate 11   see BEDOUINS

Land of the little-known kingdoms, Minaean and Sabaean, of the first millenium B.C. which were invaded by the Assyrians and Romans. From the earliest periods the country has been occupied by Semitic peoples. The Christians found refuge in the land and large numbers of Jews made it their home. It is said that the earliest Arabians lacked artistic, creative talent but by employing the artists of the countries they conquered, they developed a truly distinctive style of their own in the decorative arts and architecture. Being Moslem, the representation of living beings or animals was religiously banned. They specialized in intricate miniature patterns inlaid in wood, brass and glass and produced exquisite manuscripts and calligraphy.

1. A children's governess in a wealthy home of Trucial Oman wearing the ankle-length gandoura and the haik of black chiffon which are embroidered with gilt threads. The face veil is black. The feet of the woman, and the child in number 2, are dyed brown for color and for toughening the skin.

2. Until 12 to 14 years old, young girls of Trucial Oman may display their colorful tobes and gaudy jewelry in public but after that they must adopt the black purdah veil. This young lady's dress is of coral chiffon brocaded in gilt and her jewelry consists of many chain necklaces strung with medallions and coins, and earrings and anklets.

3. A small boy of Trucial Oman in a dark blue tobe, carrying a silver-mounted dagger in his belt. Like his elders he wears the kaffiyeh or headcloth held on the head by the agal, a decorative fillet usually of thick woolen cords wound with gold, silver and silk thread and ornamented with tufts of goat's hair. More often the agal is a hoop of goat's hair. The youngster wears blue socks and Western shoes.

4. A business man of Kuwait wearing the tobe, probably dark blue, under a Western-style jacket, and over that a dark blue cloth aba. His headcloth is secured by the goat's-hair agal.

5. A merchant of Saudi Arabia in the white linen or cotton tobe and a knitted white skullcap which is often worn under the headcloth.

6. A gentleman of Saudi Arabia in a handsome, sheer white silk kibr ornamented with gold neckband and tasseled cord worn over the tobe. Also sheer and voluminous is his headcloth of the style described in number 3.

7. A lavish silk costume in deep purple and cerise with fine embroidery. The cerise gandoura is worn over a purple robe and the color of the embroidered headcloth is also cerise.

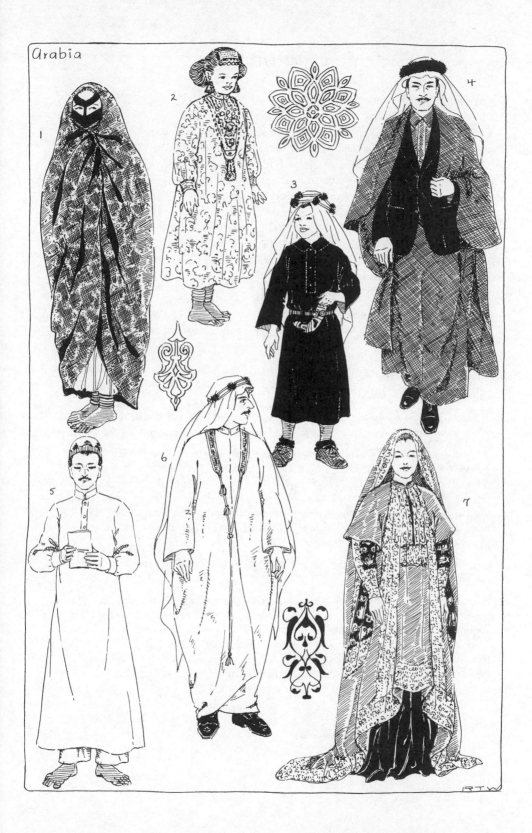

Arabia

❊ *Argentina* ❊

Plate 12

The South American Republic of Argentina occupies the eastern coast of the continent, colonization first taking place in 1536 at Buenos Aires. The livestock of the Pampa Indians consisted of llama but no cattle. In 1552, two Portuguese brothers succeeded in bringing over the Atlantic seven cows and one bull and by 1600, many cattle, sheep, goats and horses had come with the Spaniards. The gaucho or Argentine cowboy was lord of the pampas until crowded out after 1850 by the rising European immigration. His background is a mixture of Spanish, Moorish and native Indian cultures while the people are mostly Spanish in descent and language. The Roman Catholic faith is the constitutionally recognized state religion but freedom of worship is tolerated.

1. An overseer of an estancia or cattle ranch. Cloth riding jacket with white pantaloons tucked into soft leather boots. White cotton shirt with a colorful square of silk or cotton tied round his neck and a felt sombrero on his head. He carries a quirt, a short-handled riding whip with a lash of braided rawhide common in Spanish-American regions.

2. A Spanish lady of the late 19th century in a red lace gown, fringed black shawl and the ever-present fan.

3. A gaucho wearing a toga-like poncho of red wool banded with yellow and self-fringed. White cotton shirt, brown cotton pantaloons, a beige felt sombrero and leather boots.

4. A gaucho in full regalia. The chiripá is a skirt formed of a square woolen blanket wrapped round the hips and held by a heavy, elaborate silver belt. It was worn into the early 20th century. Jacket and chiripá are of red cloth, the chiripá edged with yellow. White cotton shirt and pantaloons and, very likely, a yellow neckerchief. On his arm, a woolen poncho and an ornamental quirt. The felt hat and leather boots are black. Formerly, the chiripá was worn over lace-trimmed, white cotton pantaloons with flaring open bottoms.

5. A servant in white cotton blouse, a red and black flower-printed cotton and a gay bandana round her neck.

Stirrups and spurs and a back view of a belt fashioned of silver coins, the belt holding the knife and bolas. The eighteen-inch knife, double-edged, is used for dueling and is the gaucho's only eating utensil. The bolas or boleadora is his lariat. Two balls of stone or hardwood covered with leather are attached to the ends of a rope. Held by one of the balls in the hand, it is swung over the head and let fly, hobbling the game. Gauchos of the pampas have a skillful and unerring aim.

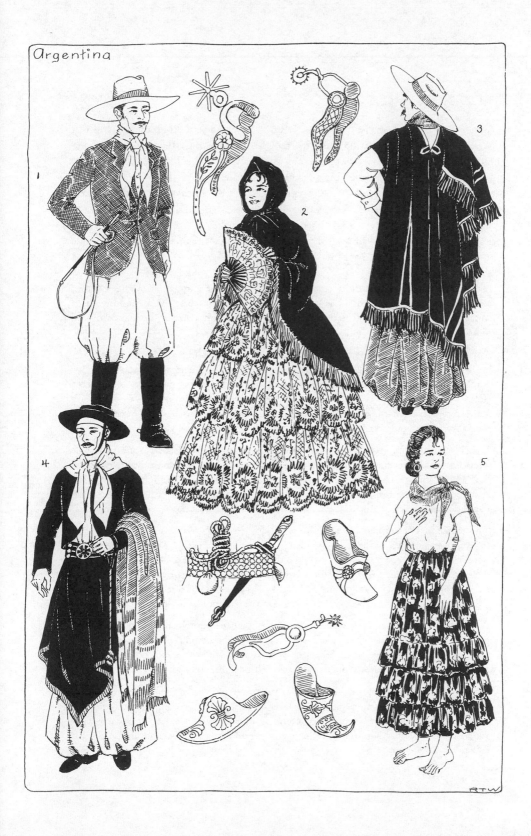

Argentina

❧ *Armenia* ❧

Plate 13   see RUSSIA

Armenia, a Soviet Socialist Republic today, was an ancient kingdom in western Asia and south Caucasia dating back to the 13th century B.C. Its history has been one of constant devastation by conquerors, the Assyrians, the Medes, the Persians; it was ruled by Alexander and his successors and then subject to Rome. The Armenians adopted Christianity as their religion, 303 A.D. They suffered persecution of the warring powers under the Arabs, Byzantines, Mongols and Turks. In the 19th century the country was partitioned between Turkey, Russia and Persia. After the Turkish defeat of World War I, the Russian sector became a Soviet Republic with the remainder taken over by Turkey.

1. A costume in orange, nasturtium red and gold. The outer garment of orange woolen cloth bordered with gold braid is girded by a wide silver belt. The headdress is a square of white silk ornamented with a gold design and the soft boots are of red moroccan leather.

2. A handsome costume of dark green cloth with gold braiding and gold-colored embroidery on the dolman jacket and chalwar or pantaloons. The white shirt is called a mintan over which is worn a combination vest and cummerbund of gold-colored cloth. His dark red tarboosh is dressed with a green silk band and a white silk scarf. Around his neck a gold chain and amulet. The babouches worn with white socks are of red moroccan leather.

3. A city woman in street costume consisting of two mantles or shawls, one of brown woolen cloth, the upper one of rose-colored heavy silk with woolen tasseled cords tied at the throat. The bonnet-shaped part is framed or wired and outlined with a ribbon sewn with silver coins which are Ottoman and old Spanish piastres, many dangling on cords.

4. The traditional Armenian bridal dress which called for heavy tissue of silk or gold thread, a long gown with train and flowing Dalmatian sleeves. The costume shown is of pea-green silk, polka-dotted with gold, over an underdress of French blue silk. A veil of white gauze is woven with a delicate flower motif in pale gold thread, a small crown of white flowers and a long face veil of gold threads. She wears her hair flowing and her peaked-toed slippers are of red moroccan leather.

5. A peasant's costume of gray woolen cloth consisting of pantaloons or chalwar, cloak and fringed blanket. Over a white shirt of heavy homespun linen is worn a red cloth bolero and a wide sash. The cap is of white felt, the socks of knitted gray yarn and the peaked-toed slippers in black with leather thongs.

6. The lady wears a tarboosh with a silver top and a brim of pale blue and deep rose velvet. Her caftan and pantaloons are of fern-green silk and the fringed silk sash of rose velvet. The chemise or blouse is of fine white cotton and worn with red moroccan leather slippers. The long silver necklace carries an amulet and silver coins.

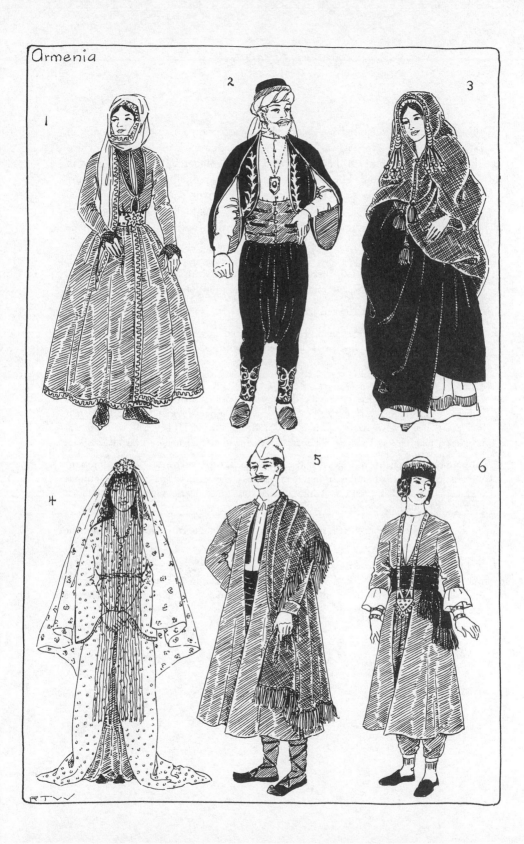

Armenia

1

2

3

4

5

6

RTW

❧ *Austria* ❧

Plate 14   see TYROL

Austria, originally inhabited by Celtic tribes, was conquered by the Romans in 14 B.C. In the Middle Ages it was part of the Holy Roman Empire and was ruled by the Hapsburgs until 1918, having formed a dual monarchy with Hungary in 1857. In 1918 Austria and Hungary became separate republics. Following many political upheavals Austria was taken over by the German Reich in 1938, invaded by Russia in 1945 and after Allied Occupation was eventually restored as an independent republic. The language is principally German and the Roman Catholic religion predominates.

1. Viennese woman in rural folk dress of silk skirt, apron with silk ties, a black velvet bodice and a shirred, chiffon skimmer with bowknot and long streamers.

2. A shirred black velvet fan-shaped hat with taffeta bows and lappets.

3. A blond maiden with hair plaited. The lace-trimmed fine white blouse was formerly the chemise. The black bodice is ornamented with silk multicolored flower embroidery. A sheer, white, lace-edged apron with braid trimming and white stockings and black slippers.

4. An 18th century costume with tall, dark green felt hat banded with ribbon of a lighter shade holding a feather. The cloth coat is ginger-colored with green collar and cuffs. Black velvet waistcoat and breeches and a wide leather belt with an embroidered motif. A varicolored silk scarf, knitted white woolen hose and black shoes.

5. A braid-bound Loden cloth jacket and suède breeches to match. A white cotton shirt with a loosely knitted pull-over in green yarn. A gay colored cravat, silver buttons and coins on a chain, knitted white woolen hose and black slippers. His "lunch basket" is a silk handkerchief of brilliant color.

6. Bonnet of golden color woven straw with white organdie frill and white organdie bow in back.

7. A bridesmaid's costume with bonnet of lace and fresh flowers and three streamers of ribbon, pale blue, pink and white. A sheer white cotton blouse, dark blue bodice and skirt with fringed shawl and frilled apron of deep sky-blue silk, the fringe a deeper shade, all bridesmaid colors.

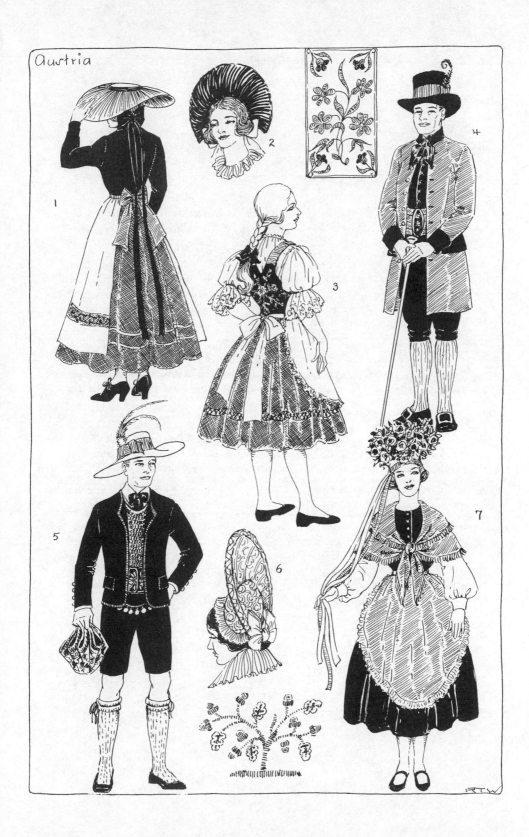

Austria

❋ *Austria* ❋

Plate 15

1. A gentleman of Burgenland, a former Austrian province, in a colorful outfit of red, black and white. Felt cap, waistcoat and leather boots are black. Scarf and breeches are of silk colored red and black. White cotton or linen shirt. The feather ornament is black, gray and white and the buttons and coins are silver. The scarfs are threaded through the armscyes.

2. The "gold hood of Linz" made of family heirloom brocade, is worn only upon special occasions, by well-to-do Linzian ladies. Of silk and gold leaf it accompanies a silk shawl and a satin apron and, as a rule, is kept in the family chest.

3. A young woman of the Wachau district wearing a family heirloom, a picture bonnet of antique gold brocade which is held secure by the tied streamers at the back of her head. Her bodice is of dark colored cloth with pleated frills, the skirt of gaily printed cotton and the apron of silk. Accessories are a white fichu, white stockings, black leather Oxfords and a sturdy straw basket.

4. Here we have the feminine silhouette of the Napoleonic Era with leg-of-mutton sleeves. The bodice is a deep purple silk with white silk fichu. A sky-blue apron partially covers a cotton skirt striped blue and white. Her headkerchief is also blue with a purple bowknot. The "market bag," a square of varicolored cotton, harmonizes with the costume. White stockings and black slippers.

5. A quaint effect, the result of the peasant combination of several colors. The fluted bonnet, sheer blouse, belt and panty ruffles are white. Bowknot, lappets and garters are deep coral. The bodice is a dull purple, the skirt wine-colored cloth bordered with the purple while the apron, also silk, is a dark green striped in black.

6. A woman of Bischofshofen wearing the early 19th century top hat in plum color banded with a ribbon to match.

7. A popular style in cloth jacket and leather shorts especially favored in black, gray or Loden green. The suspenders and wide leather belt are tooled and embroidered with the edelweiss motif in color as shown at the lower edge of the page. The shirt is white, either linen or cotton, with a colorful scarf. The large beaver felt hat with ribbon band carries tail feathers of the cock-of-the-wood but may also be ornamented with hawk wings, chamois hair plumes or even flowers.

Austria

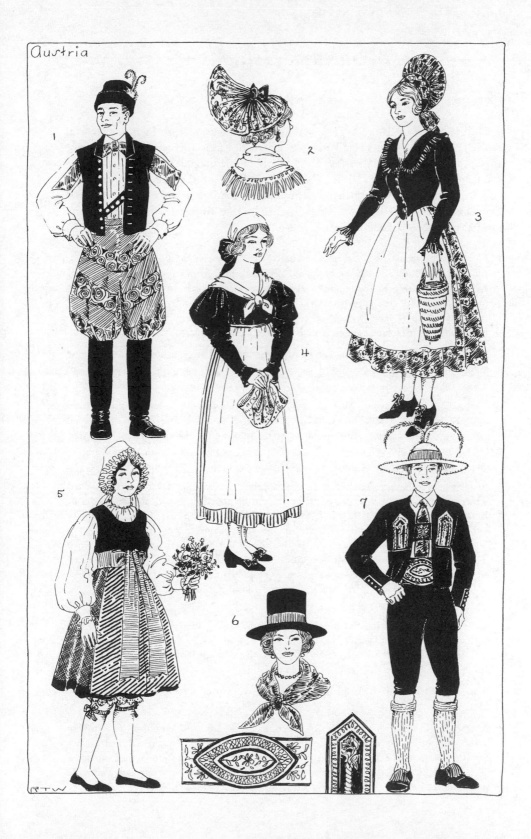

1

2

3

4

5

6

7

RTW

❧ *Balearic Islands* ❧

Plate 16

The Balearic Islands are a group in the Mediterranean Sea, Majorca, Minorca, Iviza, Formentera, Cabrera and many smaller ones near the east coast of Spain. In the 5th century B.C. they became part of the Carthaginian Empire and were conquered by Rome in 123 B.C. They were overrun by the Vandals, Byzantines and Arabs in turn until permanently conquered in the 10th century by the Ommiad Dynasty of caliphs at Cordova. Partially held by the British in the 18th century, the Balearics then became a Spanish province.

1. Man's gala costume of black breeches and black or scarlet waistcoat. Roman-striped silk cummerbund, a finely embroidered white cotton or linen shirt with a bright colored silk scarf over the shoulder. The trousers are tightly tied round the ankles by the strings of the alpargatas, the rope-soled canvas sandal of Spain and the Balearics which is now giving way to the leather shoe. The classical headcovering is the knitted barretina bonnet folded down on one side.

2. Coiffure of the young woman, her hair plaited and tied with a bowknot. A fringed and embroidered cashmere shawl and the robozilla, a flattering headkerchief of white tulle.

3. A dancer in the dress of Majorca, a black velvet skirt with a scarlet silk bodice. She also wears a style of robozilla in embroidered white batiste and a fan-shaped silk gorget, a headdress reminiscent of the 16th century. Black slippers with red heels and white stockings.

4. A young woman of Iviza in her Sunday best, her hair dressed as in number 2 and covered with a gay headkerchief in shades of yellow and orange. Over several starched white petticoats are worn skirt and bodice of red or green serge with a short apron of Roman-striped taffeta. On her feet, canvas alpargatas with turned-up toes and white stockings. Over the fringed black shawl are gold chains looped from shoulder to shoulder and held by brooches. Under the chains are coins and a large gold cross. These, the family jewels, are worn by the eldest daughter, upon her marriage passing to the next in line of unwedded daughters. The jewels are hers to wear by legal right until she marries. They serve as a sign of the family's means and of the dowry.

5. A style dating from the early 18th century of green or red serge worn over several starched white petticoats and a white cotton chemise. The sleeves are laced to the armscyes and lacings fasten the corselet. The apron tied with ribbons is of cloth with an embroidered yoke. Ruff and frilled cap are topped by a straw hat and the sandals are of canvas.

6. A black felt hat edged with shirred black velvet worn over a robozilla of embroidered silk.

7. A costume dating from the late 18th century with the apron bound with yellow braid and topped by a yoke embroidered in many colors as is the fringed yellow cashmere shawl. The felt sombrero is ornamented on the left side with a nosegay. The sleeves are buttoned to the elbow with silver buttons. The white lawn chemise shows at the neck. White stockings and canvas alpargatas complete the dress.

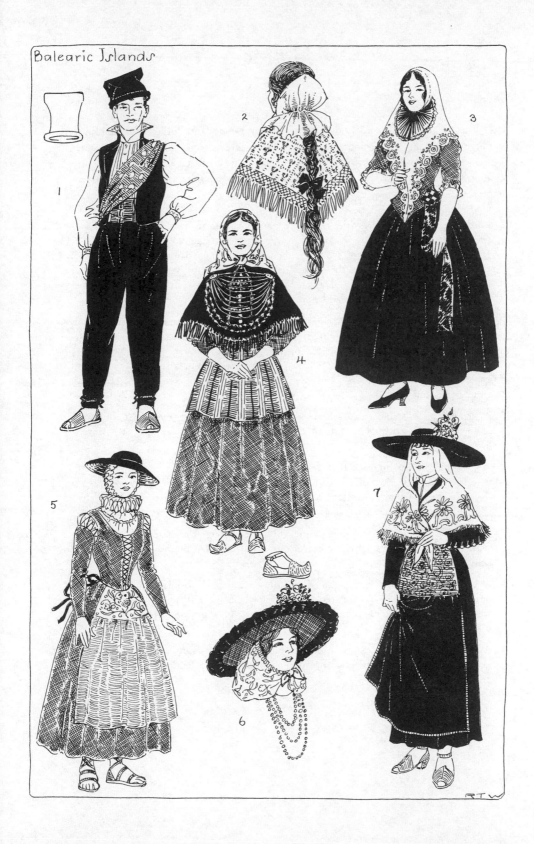

Balearic Islands

✹ *Bali* ✹

Plate 17

see INDONESIA

Bali or "Little Java" is an island of the former Netherland Indies with a Hindu civilization, having been colonized in early times direct from India. It came under Dutch domination in the early 19th century, by the turn of that century recognizing Dutch supremacy. It is now part of the Indonesian Republic. In art the Balinese excel as sculptors in gold, silver and iron work.

1. Formerly, in feminine dress the legs were always concealed by the long sarong and the bosom only covered by a cloth or towel when entering the temple. In 1955 a Bali law decreed "shirts" for women although when a woman works in the field, she is nearly always nude to the waist. In the illustration the sarong is orange with dark green motifs, a yellow and green border and a green sash. Artistically draped is the cream-colored cotton headdress.

2. The training of a Balinese dancing girl begins when five years old, her dancing career ending from twelve to fourteen years of age when she returns to village life. The dances are centuries old, based upon mythology, folklore and history, never varying. This costume is of gold on black with a wide gold sash. The crown and collarette are of polychromed, perforated buffalo leather, the crown filled in with fresh frangipani blossoms.

3. A temple ballet dancer with polychromed tiara built up of two rows of paper feathers and the outer row of fresh flowers. The collarette is also of polychromed leather.

4. A handsome sarong in dark blue cotton with motifs of a lighter shade tied over a waistband of pink cloth. Today, the bare torso has almost entirely given way to the wearing of the white cotton Western shirt. The headdress is composed of two bandanas, one white and one colored.

5. The white cotton Western shirt worn with the sarong, the latter of red cotton with cream floral motifs, a yellow border and a red sash. On the head is tied a white cotton bandana.

6. A nine-year old ballet dancer. All blacks shown are really brilliant silk hammered with gold leaf. Crown and collarette are of gilded buffalo leather, the crown holding fresh frangipani blossoms. Underskirt and fan are of a muted raspberry tone with pale rose motifs.

7. A colorful fête day costume of silk, the sarong black with orange flower motifs. The kabaya or jacket is of mauve with black and orange flowers and the cummerbund is orange and gold.

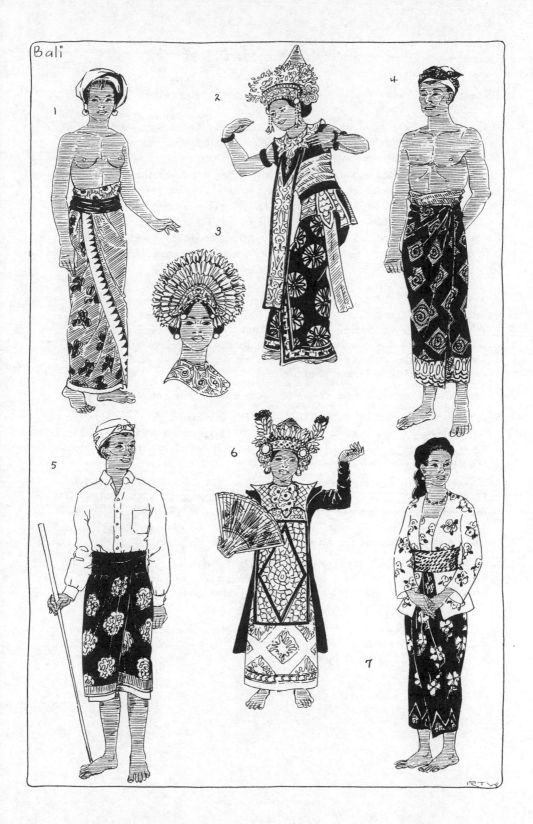

Bali

1

2

3

4

5

6

7

RTW

❧ *Barbary States* ❧

Plate 18   see ALGERIA, BEDOUINS, MOROCCO

The Barbary States of Morocco, Algeria, Tunisia and Tripolitania were overrun by the Vandals in the 5th century, by Byzantium in the 6th century and by the Moors in the 7th. They became independent Moslem states known as the Barbary States, a corruption of the word "Berberie" meaning the land of the Berber. The origin of these white-skinned people is not known. European penetration began with the Portuguese taking over Ceuta in 1415, Tripoli conquered by the Spanish in 1509–1511 and Algiers in 1541. Tripoli fell to the Turks in 1551. The United States War with Tripoli in 1801–1805 and with Algiers in 1815 and the British bombardment in 1816 put an end to the piracy and tribute carried on by the Barbary States.

1. A member of the Ouled-Naïl tribe in the Atlas Mountains and a dancer in Algeria cafés. An over-elaborate costume with underdress of pale blue cotton, a Nile green yoke and a white cotton tunic. The white mantle is lined with black goatskin. Accessories are black slippers with blue stockings, a jeweled gold tiara, coins and bracelets. Costumes 1 and 4 are not cut and sewn but are draped lengths of cloth held by a ribbon around the neck and often a belt.

2. and 6. Hands, feet and ankles of a Berber woman stenciled or tattooed with henna.

3. A spahi or native cavalryman of Tripolitania. His costume is white, sky blue and red. A blue wool bolero edged with red over the long-sleeved, full-length tobe of white cotton sashed with red. Two barracanos, the Bedouin cloth covers, one red, the other blue, and black leather shoes.

4. A Berber woman goes unveiled, has property rights, can divorce easily and remarry. Over the white chemise, a length of cloth of indigo blue cotton with a fold across the chest and a blue self girdle. Headgear consists of a tarboosh draped with blue and worn over a red and yellow headcloth. The lady, who has come to the village well for water, wears bracelets, brooches and a necklace.

5. A Tunisian costume in three cotton fabrics, a red and yellow stripe, plain white and a multicolored print on a white ground. A red sash with beaded tassel. The headdress is yellow with a beaded ornament and headkerchief, added to which she wears a beaded necklace, brooches and a chatelaine.

7. The personal servant of a Moroccan chief in a brown and white striped cotton kibr worn over the white cotton tobe. His turban is of white cotton and he carries a silver-sheathed dirk, his ever-present arm.

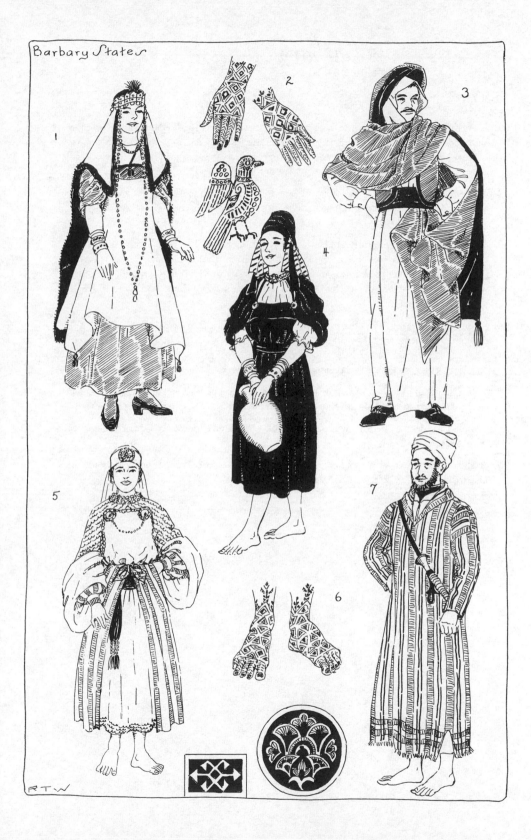

Barbary States

RTW

❧ *Barbary States* ❧

Plate 19

1. A member of the spahi police bodyguard of the governor of Tripolitania. Sky blue cloth bolero jacket with a red stripe on the sleeves and red and green cuff points. Draped red and white barracanos. The garment is the long-sleeved, long-skirted desert shirt or kamis. Red fez, brown leather sandals and his sword.

2. A Berber woman of Tripolitania in an interesting headcovering of indigo blue cotton tied in back over a tarboosh. The headcloth is also cotton, red striped with yellow.

3. A Tuareg in his gracefully draped cloak or k'sa of indigo blue cloth, cotton or wool, which is simply a piece of fabric about six yards long which he wears over the long shirt called a kumya and pantaloons. Turban and fold around neck are white and the luxurious woolen scarf is striped in gray, blue and white. Knob sandals on his feet.

4. A city-bred girl of Tripolitania in a costume of orchid-colored satin brocade for the undergarment with the draped piece of heavy beige satin striped in wine red. The latter is secured by a belt and shoulder bands. A necklace of gold coins, bracelets, earrings and jeweled plaques will be her dowry.

5. A shepherd of Tunisia in white cotton carrying a burnous or blanket of woolen cloth. The turban is cotton in mauve and a wine red plaid. Yellow leather babouches.

6. A veiled Moslem woman in white cotton haik and yellow moroccan leather babouches with turned-up toes.

7. A shoe worn by an Arab soldier of Libya. Of heavy leather, rough side out, with an ornamental stop to keep the trouser leg in place.

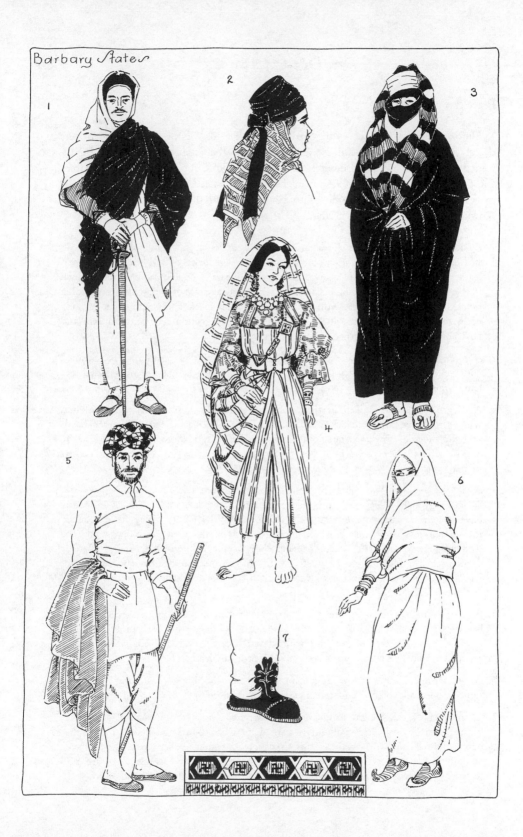

Barbary States

❧ *Bedouins* ❧

Plate 20

The Bedouins are people who lead a nomadic life, living principally in the desert. Today's Bedouins comprise a large part of the Arabian population. In ancient times they roamed the deserts of Egypt and Syria, spreading to Mesopotamia and Chaldea. The conquest of Africa in the 7th century A.D. opened up new regions so that today they are to be met with from Persia to the Atlantic and from the Kurdistan Mountains to the Sudan.

1. A desert patrolman of the Jordanian Army in a caftan of khaki cloth, the long sleeves lined with white cotton. Straps and cartridge belts of red morocco leather, leather quirt and a dirk in a silver sheath. He wears a double kaffiyeh, one which is the distinguishing mark of his status, a square headcloth of red with white polka dots, the other a white one with tufted cotton. The black agal carries the insignia of his company. Under the caftan, he wears the white cotton tobe and trousers and boots of soft cordovan leather.

2. A young prince in a sheer and protective tobe over his kihr of vermilion silk trimmed with yellow braid. He wears the white kaffiyeh with black agal. Black tasseled ties hang from the neck of the tobe.

3. A Negro girl from El Teb in the Sudan. A graceful, simple robe, the gandoura, which might be brown, black or dark blue. Two necklaces, one of amber beads and the other of silver in the motif shown to her left. Her hair is in short, tight braids with a silver roundel on her forehead, silver hoops in her ears and pearls in her nostrils.

4. A Tuareg in his white cotton turban. The Tuaregs are related to the Berbers and ancient Egyptians. They were originally warriors but today, under French influence, have become herders and own the finest camels in the desert. They have retained their Hamitic speech and alphabet. Though Moslem, the men go veiled while the women go unveiled. The litham or face cloth is the distinguishing mark of their dress in black, indigo blue or white, worn as a protection against sun and sand. That of the nobles is black or blue, white for commoners, hence the terms "black" or "white" Tuareg.

5. An Arab girl of Cyrenaica who covers her face when in public. She wears earrings, bracelets, fillet and coins of gold and a mark of tattooing on her chin. Her dress is black over a bodice of red and white lawn. Leather belt and silk tasseled sash are white, and her boots are of soft brown cordovan leather.

6. A woman of Hausa in the Sudan in a handsomely draped headdress, her hair tightly rolled and plaited and ornamented with gold coins.

7. A member of the Desert Mounted Police serving under the French flag. Berber, Tuareg and Moorish, he is stunningly garbed in white cotton and black. The leather boots and turban are black, the turban of black cotton. When necessary he will veil his face to the eyes as protection against sand and sun. His feet, too, are protected by a brown solution to toughen them. He carries a gun, dirk and quirt.

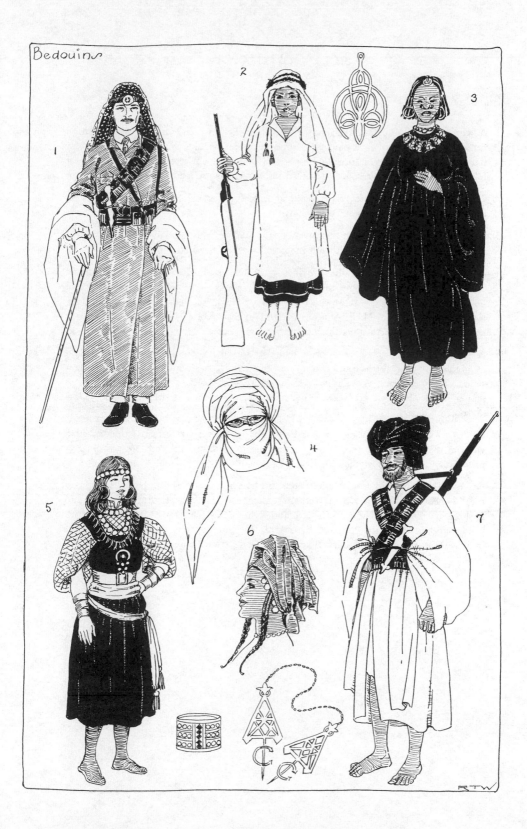

Bedouins

❧ *Bedouins* ❧

Plate 21

1. A woman of the Kabyles of Algeria or Tunisia, a Berber race dating from prehistoric times. Many of them have blue eyes, ruddy complexion and wavy brown hair. Her hair is dressed in heavy turned-up braids. The pantaloon costume is a mixture of fabrics, colors and jewelry, girdled with a sash of Roman-striped silk.

2. The coiffure of a daughter of a sheik, a princess about 14 years of age, her hair puffed and dressed with gold ornaments.

3. A Tuareg trader in a white cotton k'sa and indigo blue turban and veil. Broad sandals of cordovan leather with red moroccan leather. See Plate 19—note 3.

4. A dancer of Ouled-Naïl of the Province of Alger in Algeria. With a tattoo mark on her forehead, her costume comprises several fabrics of varied colors, jewelry and gold coins. The jewelry represents her dowry which she herself has amassed by living for a time in Mediterranean ports. Having accomplished that, she returns home to marriage and a quiet life among her own people.

5. A sheik's costume, the kibr of fine white cotton marked with an invisible plaid in gold and silver threads and worn over the kamis or shirt and trousers of plain white. The headdress or kaffiyeh is sheer white with black agal. He carries a gun and in his leather belt a silver-sheathed dirk. The soft slippers are of red or yellow moroccan leather.

6. A Tuareg turban of solid indigo blue and indigo blue with a Roman stripe accented with a fold of pure white. The Tuaregs avoid brightly colored dress, adhering principally to deep shades of blue and black and white.

7. Except for hands and feet, Moslem local custom requires that in public a woman must be covered. This Arabian woman returning from market wears the veil and a sheer black haik. Her dress is red and yellow, her pantaloons red edged with yellow and her feet are protected by a kind of gaiter of soft, black leather. Pieces of jewelry with green and dark blue enamels and coral stones.

Bedouins

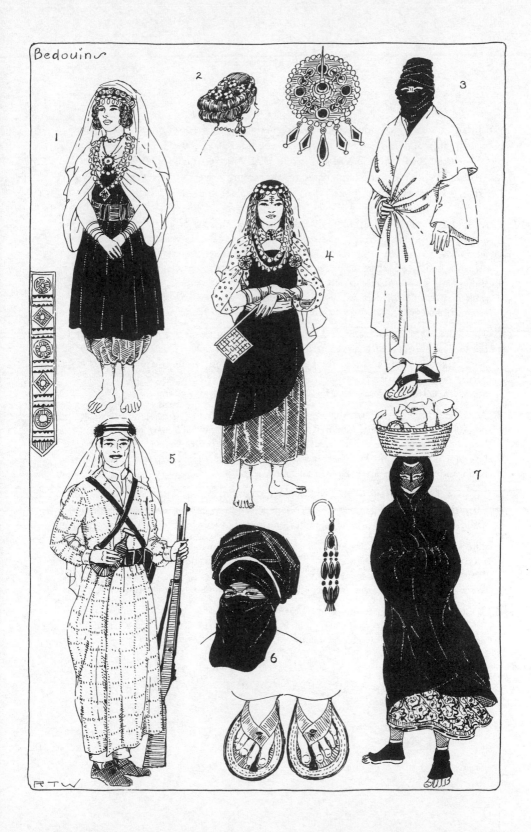

RTW

❊ *Bhutan* ❊

Plate 22

Bhutan, a semi-independent country, formerly a British protectorate, is situated between Tibet and India in the center of the Himalayas, the highest mountains on the earth. British relations dated from 1772. Mistreatment of British subjects led to an invasion in 1865 and parts of the country were annexed to India. A hereditary maharajah rules subject to the approval of the Indian Government.

1. A Bhutanese woman in a brilliantly colored homespun robe of coral, gray and black draped over an undergarment and held securely by a kera or waistband. Over it she wears a short woolen jacket and shawl. The shawl is an important accessory in the dress of both sexes, there being an appropriate shawl for each and every occasion. Individuals always greet each other by exchanging white shawls. Red shawls denote rank at gala affairs. Men, women and children wear their coarse, heavy, black hair cropped short and usually go barefoot, even in the snow.

2. The schoolboy's costume is of dark blue homespun worn over a white undergarment, the long sleeves of which are turned back as protective cuffs. This masculine robe is belted tightly round the waist, the bloused upper section forming a roomy front and back where one carries possessions necessary for the day. The white cotton breeches are worn only upon occasions, this occasion being a royal wedding.

3. A prince's bride in her wedding dress of heavy taupe silk woven with flowers in white, rose and pale blue. Under it is a long-sleeved, pink silk garment. The apron is of multi-colored hand-loomed silk. Around her neck she wears a jeweled charm box of ivory, coral and turquoise beads and stones. Her hair is dressed in a coronet braid and on her feet are open-toed silk sandals.

4. Like the boy's dress above, this is also a long robe drawn up and belted into a real carry-all to hold just about anything, food, a drinking cup or even a cooking pot. Of linen or cotton cloth printed in yellow and red and worn with white undergarment.

5. The lama is a monk or teacher of Buddhism and many men and boys join the monastery to receive state support. The traditional dedication of a child from each family to the religion is today being discouraged. A length of vermilion cotton cloth is wrapped over a sleeveless garment of yellow silk bordered with vermilion bands.

6. A Bhutanese official in formal dress wearing the red shawl signifying rank. His robe is of brocaded silk in white and yellow with motifs in red and dark green and, underneath, the usual white garment.

Bhutan

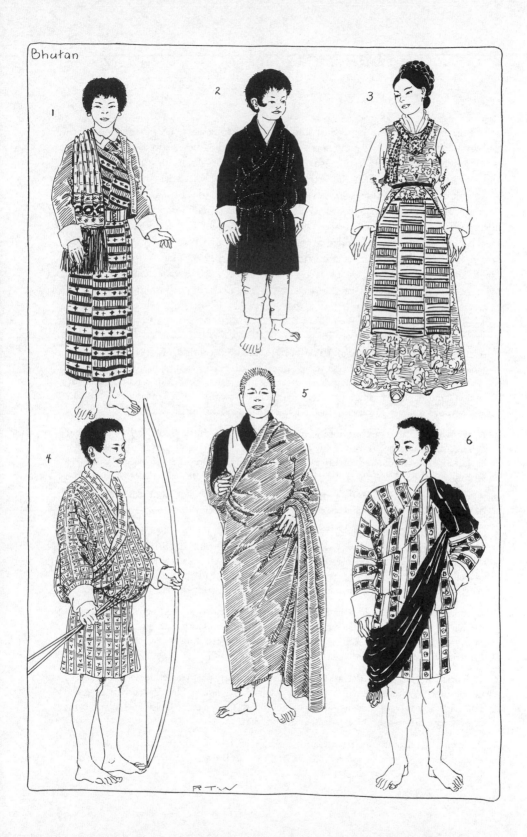

❧ *Bible Lands: Israel and Jordan* ❧

Plate 23

From earliest times the land once known as Palestine has been invaded and settled by peoples from the south, north and west and has been successively part of
many foreign empires. Palestine was conquered by the Arabs in the 7th century
and except for the period in the 12th century when the Crusaders held Jerusalem,
it was under Moslem rule until World War I when the British conquered the
state. In 1939 the British approved Palestine as a national home of the Jews but
during World War II conflict arose between Jews, Arabs and the British. In 1947
the United Nations recommended a partition of Palestine between Jews and Arabs
which finally took place in an armistice agreement in 1949. The partition running
north and south cut the City of Jerusalem in half. The Transjordan Arabs took
over the old city and Israel captured the new city, declaring it part of the state of
Israel in 1949. So, as it stands today, Jews and Arabs are still technically at war
with each other.

1. A peasant farmer or fellah of Palestine. His costume consists of the striped cotton
   tobe, over a kamis or cotton shirt and the aba of coarse homespun or camel's-hair
   cloth. Upon his head, the kaffiyeh, a striped white cotton headcloth and a goat's-hair
   agal. Comfortable papushes protect his feet. The sword is for possible use should
   a marauder appear, meanwhile he keeps watch upon his field workers.

2. A woman of Palestine carrying water. Her dress or khurkeh of dark blue linen,
   a long, straight robe, is belted by a sash of varicolored cashmere. Bodice and edge
   of jacket are embroidered in brilliant colors. Both sides of the skirt are slashed revealing an undergarment; on her head, the khalak of white cotton cloth.

3. A patriarch or scribe of Palestine wearing a velour tarboosh and silk snood, not
   unlike a fashionable feminine headdress in the present era.

4. A bride of a village of Judea wearing the khurkeh and her wedding bonnet, the
   feature of which is the dowry, a heavy, solid row of gold and silver coins forming
   the outer frame of the bonnet. Her dress is of silk, yellow striped with red, a yoke
   of yellow and red plaid, sleeves of solid orange color and underskirt of vivid green.
   All the embroidery, done in many colors, is the handwork of the young woman.

5. A young woman of Bethlehem or Nazareth dressed up in an heirloom of her grandmother's. A caftan of hand-spun, Tyrian purple silk and wrought gold with a wide
   sash tied in front, the ends weighted with fat tassels. She wears a red tarboosh
   banded with red silk over a gay silk headcloth.

6. A Christian girl of Jerusalem wearing the headgear of the Bethlehem costume, a
   tarboosh with white veil which indicates a married woman. Her tarboosh is of green
   felt with red velvet to which is sewn gold and silver coins. Gold and silver coins
   also dangle from the chain attached to her hat.

7. A Jewish gentleman of Jerusalem in an aba of heavy silk in apricot color worn
   over a cotton caftan of yellow striped in brown. Brown fur cap, white socks and
   black leather peak-toed shoes.

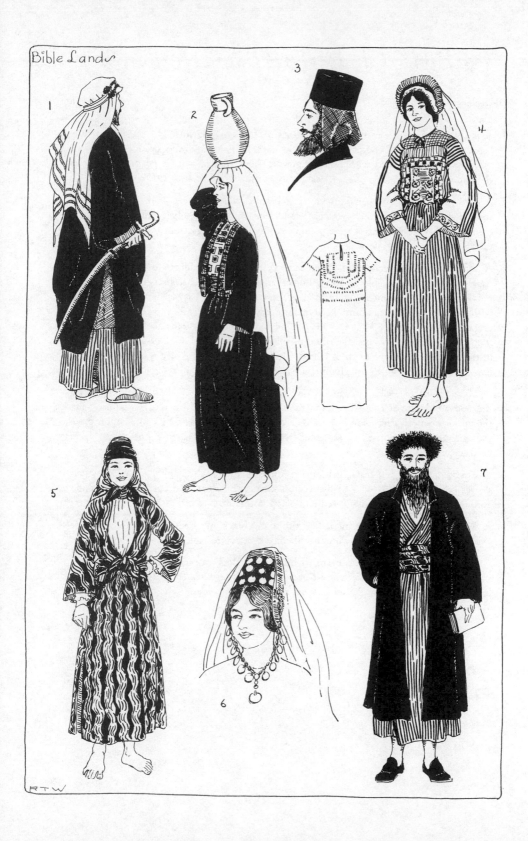

Bible Lands

RTW

❧ *Bible Lands: Israel and Jordan* ❧

Plate 24

1. A sheik, director of a convent in Palestine for Moslem pilgrims. His aba is surely a "coat of many colors" striped unevenly in dark blue, purple and orange on a pure white ground and lined with peacock green. The caftan is a dark purple worn over the kamis or white cotton shirt. Black papushes and white socks. (1920's)

2. A Moslem matron of a small town of Palestine. Her bonnet of silk with a plum-colored silk headkerchief has two chaplets formed of gold and silver coins. Such a rich bonnet often weighs eight or nine pounds. A large coin hangs from the chain attached to the cap.

3. A married Moslem woman of Bethlehem wearing the Bethlehem dress or khurkeh usually made in dark blue and red. Bodice, undersleeves and trouser-shaped skirt are red with a pink cummerbund sash. The short jacket and back panel are dark blue with colorful silk thread and bead embroidery. Over the tall bonnet, shatweh, is draped the veil called a khalak. This feminine silhouette has come to light on figures found on vases recently unearthed in the Holy Land and which carbon-14 dating places in the century before the birth of Christ. Here, no doubt, is the origin of the medieval hennin carried back to Europe by the Crusaders.

4. A Moslem girl of Palestine wearing the barracan, a length of cloth wrapped round the body and drawn over the head and shoulders. Originally of coarse camlet, that shown in the illustration is of heavy silk, red striped with black. The white cotton piece over the left shoulder serves as handkerchief, napkin or whatever one might have need of.

5. A Christian girl in her festal Palestine costume of oyster-white linen with Dalmatian sleeves embroidered in red and black cross-stitch. The skirt is draped trouser-fashion and held by a crushed girdle of red and black cashmere.

6. A Moslem woman wearing instead of the thick, black mandeel or face veil a cooler one of thin, figured muslin with either the black or white haik.

7. A Christian shepherd of Bethlehem in his striped cloth caftan over the white cotton kamis or shirt. His accessories consist of the white cotton kaffiyeh with goat's-hair agal, leather belts and pouch and leather shoes with turned-up toes.

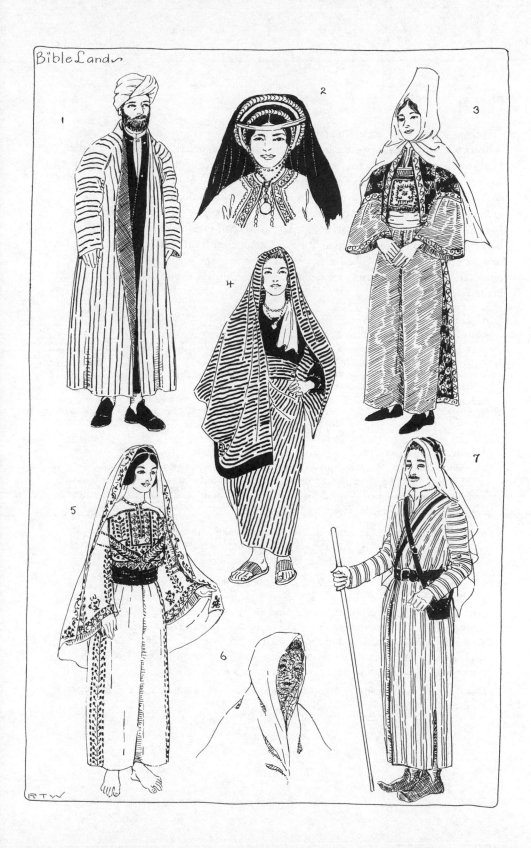

BibleLand

✻ *Bolivia* ✻

Plate 25

Bolivia, in the west central part of South America, is the land of the Aymara Indians who already possessed a high culture when conquered by the Incas in the 13th and 14th centuries. They became one of the most important components of the Inca Empire. They achieved independence from Spain in 1825 and called a congress to declare the state a republic. The name Bolivia is based upon that of the great South American liberator, Bolivar. The greater part of the population is Indian with a foreign population of pure and half-caste Spanish. The official language is Spanish and in religion, Roman Catholicism leads although other forms of worship are permitted. The Indians continue to spin the yarn and weave the colorful fabrics of their wearing apparel made of cotton, linen and wool and handmade at home.

1. A young mother of Tiahuanaco carrying her baby in a red woolen shawl called a rebozo. With a green woolen skirt she wears a white linen blouse. Her very odd hat is of blue cloth draped over a box-shaped cap underneath, the whole resembling a parlor lamp. Her hair is dressed in two braids.

2. Bolivians adore fantastic fiesta hats. We came upon this beauty in research dated 1908 and again in the 1950's. Such creations are treasured. The ostrich plumes, white with black tips, are procured from the birds which roam the Chaco Desert and mounted on a wicker frame, making a very light bonnet.

3. A native of Sucre, the constitutional capital of Bolivia. His leather helmet, a family heirloom, resembles the morion of the Spanish conquistadors. He wears white linen breeches and a small woolen poncho striped red, yellow and black, and carries a folded woolen serape or blanket. Around his waist a hand-loomed pouch in red and yellow and on his feet homemade leather sandals.

4. A farmer's wife in a blue cotton blouse with red yoke and cuffs banded with white braid embroidery. The skirt is red cotton with brown braid embroidery. Over the coiffure of two braids she wears a beige felt hat with brown ribbon band.

5. A Bolivian miss in her church-going frock of tucked lawn shirt and a bodice of velvet and lace. With her hair in braids, she wears a white straw derby. It is odd that the hard felt hat which originated in England in the mid-nineteenth century for the "upper class" has, since the beginning of our century, been the favorite headpiece of the Chola Indians, especially among the women. Of course, its wearing qualities are responsible for its becoming so. Black, brown and beige are the favored colors. The topper too, was adopted, but in straw. So very un-Indian!

Most of the fabrics worn by the peasant class, such as cotton, linen and wool are hand-woven at home.

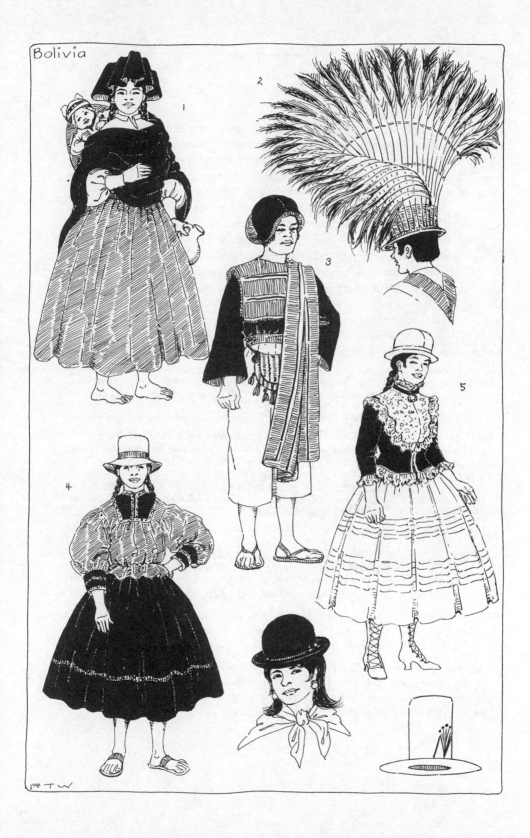

Bolivia

❧ *Brazil* ❧

Plate 26

Brazil, the largest country in South America, lies to the east of the Andes, its coastline of about 4,000 miles bordering the Atlantic. A Spaniard claimed discovery of Brazil in 1500 although it had been allotted to Portugal by treaty in 1494. There followed settlements under a system of hereditary captaincies by the Spanish in 1552, by the French in 1555 and by the Dutch in 1650 to 1654. The productions of minerals, gold, silver and diamonds, sugar and coffee in the 18th century caused constant friction. In 1750, Madrid recognized expanded Portuguese boundaries. In 1891, Brazil became the United States of Brazil. Freedom of worship exists though the country is largely Catholic, and the language is Portuguese.

"Costume" to Brazilians means "Carnival", the yearly three-day pre-Lenten frolic in which costumed merrymakers, both rich and poor, dance and perform in the streets and hotel ballrooms. Dress ranges from the frugal homemade bit to the most lavish outfits costing enormous sums of money. The mummers plan their raiment and floats all year and after the great event is over, start planning at once for the next pre-Lenten Carnival.

1. A Turkish-inspired costume of black velvet with gold braid, red sash and red slippers. The gorgeous white satin turban carries a red panache and a sparkling cabochon.

2. A striking gown with grass green taffeta bodice and tunic over a dazzlingly figured skirt of orange and green silk. The lady wears a gold baldric and ropes of large pearls. Her trim turban is of bronze silk with a cabochon and her slippers are also bronze.

3. One of a "blocos" or group of workmen who dress in feminine garb and parade together. This participant because of his bead necklaces looks more like an African potentate. The robe is of bright dark blue and white satin with bands of black satin. His turban in lamé is gun-metal gray and his sandals are of the same color.

4. A Negress of the late 19th century in traditional dress, a costume that could very well pass for a Paris couturière model today. The dress is either black or dark blue with a border of red and the poncho of wool striped red and yellow. The turban fabrics are wool or cotton in white with silver and red and yellow stripes.

5. A drummer in a black silk shirt checked with variegated pale tinted squares, dark blue breeches and red slippers. He wears a straw sombrero and a red neckerchief and his drum is colored yellow with red.

6. A "lady pirate" in a castellated outfit of white satin blouse and black velvet breeches. A black leather belt with silver buckle and the important dirk. A black felt hat, black leather wristlets, modern black boots of leather, rubber or synthetic, all properly tagged with skull and crossbones.

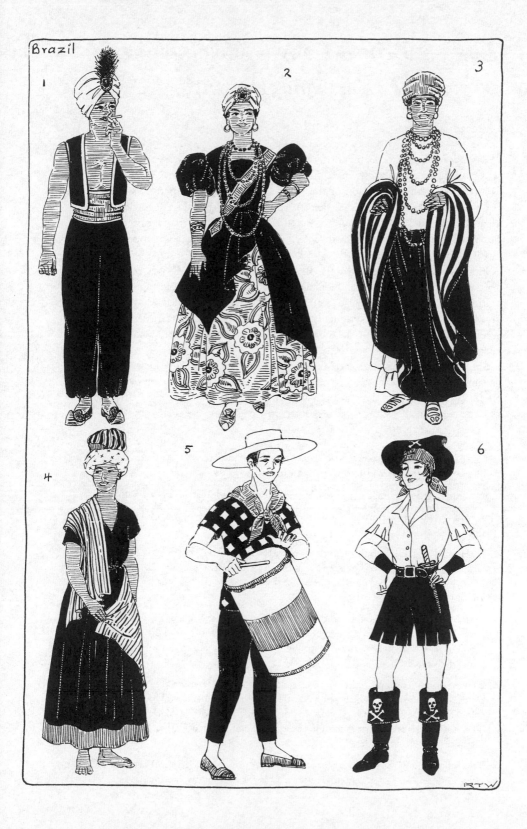

Brazil

❋ British Crown Colonies ❋
Past and Present

Plate 27

Barbados, though probably discovered in the 16th century by the Portuguese, was claimed by the English in 1605 and was taken over by the Crown in 1663. It is now part of the Federation of the West Indies. Its chief export is sugar.

Cyprus, in the eastern Mediterranean, was colonized by the Phoenicians and ancient Greeks, and has been raided, captured and ruled by many eastern empires, lastly the Turks. Made a Crown Colony in 1914, it is now a republic within the British Commonwealth.

Hong Kong was occupied by the British in 1839, and in 1841 was ceded to them by the Chinese. It was severely bombed and then occupied by the Japanese 1941–45.

Malta is the chief island of a group known as the Maltese Islands formerly constituting a British colony. Originally it was a Phoenician and Carthaginian colony. Malta developed a powerful naval base in the 19th century. It became an independent member of the Commonwealth in 1964.

Singapore was an important Malay city in the 13th century. Destroyed by the Javanese in the 14th century, it remained in ruins until refounded by the British in 1819. By developing a great port and trade center it became the "Crossroads to the Far East". In 1946 it became a British Crown Colony. See Plate 68.

1. A young woman of Cyprus in a beautifully gold-embroidered black velvet bolero combined with a full skirt of black and white checked soft silk. A sheer white cotton blouse completes the costume worn with black suède shoes.

2. A Chinese girl of Hong Kong wearing an effective shade hat of woven bamboo.

3. A young lady of Cyprus in a smart red felt fez enhanced by an elegant, long black silk tassel.

4. In Hong Kong the popular Chinese "everyday-work-a-day" outfit of navy blue cotton jacket and slacks is worn by men, women and children. Here, we have a picturesque shade hat of orange-colored straw beflounced with a deep frill of blue muslin. The shoes are blue and white, probably canvas.

5. Many women of Singapore and Hong Kong wear the cheongsam or "Shanghai gown." The model shown is of black and white polka dot foulard with white silk bindings and frog fasteners. This young woman wears a slip under her sheath and white canvas sandals.

6. The Barbados Harbor Police wear a good-looking and comfortable uniform devised by the British in 1748 which set the pattern for most other naval powers in cut and color, hence the term "navy blue." In blue and white with a black silk neckerchief. The straw hat has a white washable cover, the silver-buckled leather belt is brown and the shoes are black leather.

7. The huke, a long, black cloth cloak of Moorish origin which is still worn by Maltese older women. Very often, as in Central Europe, it is a family heirloom.

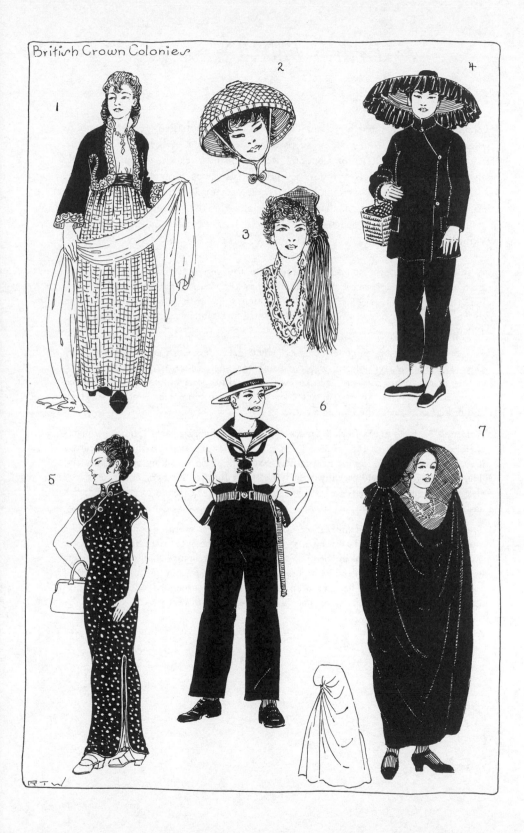

British Crown Colonies

✳ *British Folk Dress* ✳

Plate 28

Established and patented merchant firms of London sold their goods in public, crying their wares in front of their shops or while walking in the street from the 15th century on. The "cries of London" were a distinct feature and it was said, really became a concert of harmony. Eventually, as shops grew larger and more affluent, the pedlars' cries were stifled. An ordinance of 1839 banned all kinds of criers in the streets, singers, pedlars and especially the fish women who sold fish of doubtful freshness. The pedlars always wore a hat, even as they do today when working in public.

1. A Billingsgate fish woman. All fish brought to the port of London had to be sold from the Billingsgate market. This feminine hawker wears a red cloak and a black felt hat over a white headkerchief. White cotton tunic with a yellow fichu, a blue cotton apron and a brown cloth skirt. White stockings and black leather shoes. Early 19th century.

2, 4, 5. A family of London costermongers in their gala dress worn at Epsom on Derby Day. The word costermongers was the name for apple-sellers in past times. These clothes of the 1930's are sewn and covered with white pearl buttons, thus the name "pearlies" as a group. An extravagant panache of ostrich plumes in white, rose, green and orange ornaments the feminine hat.

3. A farmer in his "smock-frock." Smock was the Anglo-Saxon word for a woman's chemise dating back to the camise of the early medieval period. In the 13th century it evolved into the working garment of both sexes, taking on smocking and embroidery. The smocking stitch held the tiny pleats together, a form of stitchery which produced elasticity for fit and fullness for ease. The man's smock was made of homespun, flax and hemp and the woman's of linen.

6. The "milk girl" who sold milk from dawn to ten in the morning and again in the afternoon up to six o'clock. By an act of Parliament she was permitted to add one third water to the milk. With her red skirt she wears a mauve blouse and panniers with a yellow fichu. Headkerchief and apron are of white muslin and the felt hat and leather shoes are black. The cans of pewter or tin are suspended on leather straps attached to the wooden yoke across her shoulders. Early 19th century.

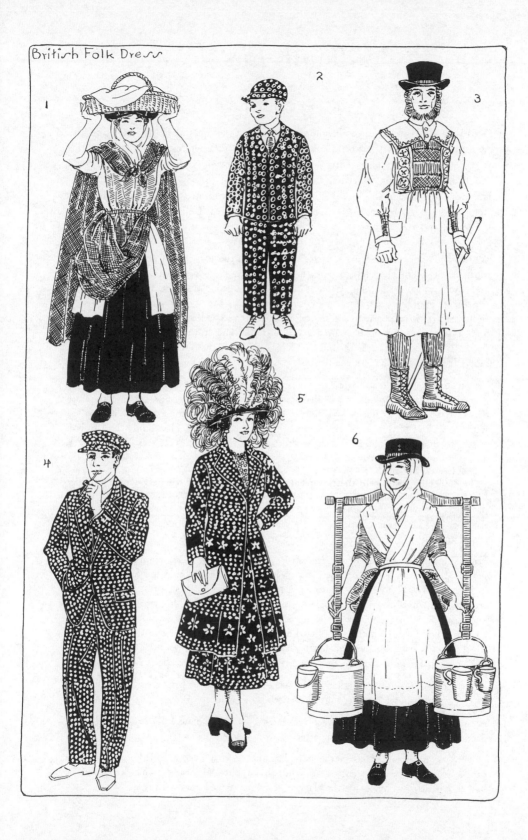

British Folk Dress

❧ *British Isles* ❧

Plate 29

Great Britain is made up of England, the largest part, bounded by Wales on the west and Scotland on the north, which were once independent kingdoms. Wales was conquered in the 13th century and Scotland was joined to England in 1603 when the Scottish king inherited the English throne.

Ireland, once part of the kingdom, was granted dominion status as the Irish Free State in 1921, and, except for six counties in northern Ireland, became an independent republic in 1949.

1. A Scottish woman in her mantle, cloak or blanket, the older form of Highland dress worn until 1740. The plaid or breacan-feile was a piece of tartan, two yards wide and four to six yards long. It was doubled, wrapped round the waist, belted and drawn up over the head. Known more commonly as the "belted plaid," the drawing shows tan cloth striped with red, a yellow skirt striped with red with bodice of green and a white muslin fichu secured by a brooch. The leather belt has a long and decorative silver tongue. Silver buckled shoes are worn with green stockings and the lady's hair is plaited and ribbon-tied.

2. The medieval uniform still worn by the Yeomen of the Guard and the Warders of the Tower of London. Bright red cloth tunic, breeches and hose have been worn since the 15th century with black and yellow braiding and gold emblazonry. The pleated white lawn ruff of the period and a black beaver hat with red, black and white ribbon cockades. Red garters and black leather shoes with red and white rosettes. White gloves, a sword and gold-tasseled lance.

3. Such a hooded cloak as this Irish woman of the 1940's wears is very often a family heirloom, sometimes richly embroidered. Of black cloth, it reveals its Moorish origin of the period when the Saracens ruled Spain. The huke, as it was called in Central Europe, was worn for centuries, finally ending up as the red cloak or "cardinal" of the 18th century, and the "Kerry" cloak in Ireland.

4. Highland dress worn during the English Prohibition Act of 1746, banning the kilt and plaid. The breacan-feile hung from the shoulders in back enabling the wearer to wrap it round his waist to hide the principal features of his Scottish dress. The law was repealed in 1782. Brown tweed jacket and sporran with light blue tweed breacan-feile and kilt. The shirt is of fine white muslin with lawn and lace cravat and the waistcoat in shades of brown and red. Red knitted woolen hose, brown leather baldric and shoes and gilt trim, buckles and buttons. The Highland "blue bonnet" of wool with a red pompon carries a sprig of native evergreen which indicates the wearer's clan.

5. A little girl of Wales wearing her grandmother's glossy beaver hat over a frilled lingerie cap. A fringed shawl over her muslin blouse and a plaid apron over a dark skirt.

6. A small Scotsman in a brown tweed jacket and a fringed plaid kilt. Scotch cuarans of deerskin with leather thong cross-gartering over woolen hose.

7. A young woman of Wales in the tall black beaver hat over a frilled white lingerie cap. Her guimpe and apron are of white lawn but the large kerchief is silk. The bodice is black combined with a black and white striped cotton skirt.

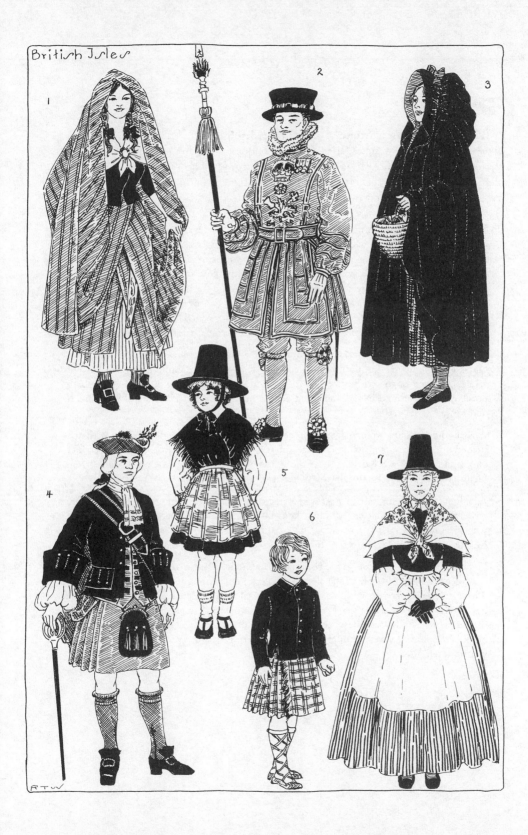

British Isles

❧ *Bulgaria* ❧

Plate 30

Bulgaria, a mainly agricultural country bordering on the Black Sea, has had, like the other Balkan states, a history of conquest and division alternated with periods of independence. It is now a Communist republic. The people are predominantly Slavic and belong to the Greek Orthodox faith, with some Moslems reflecting a former period of Turkish rule.

1. Until recently, the wearing of "store clothes" was either a sign of indolence or lack of ability. Bulgarian women worked the hemp and flax seeds from ground through to spinning, weaving, cutting and sewing of all the garments of the family. The white braided and embroidered dark cloth overdress permits the display of a fine, beautifully handworked white chemise. The cloth belt is fastened by a heavy silver buckle called a pafti. A shamiya or headcloth of white, red or green tied over the crown of the head denotes a maiden and when tied under the chin, a married woman. Carbatines or leather bottines are laced over white woolen stockings. The parasol is of white muslin.

2. A peasant's costume in black and white. The white serge breeches are braided in black, and the homespun black cloth, décolleté jacket or aba is embroidered in red and white. The vest of the white linen shirt is also done in red and white. A wide, plaid-bordered cummerbund in red and black adds a bit more color. His sheepskin tarboosh and leather shoes are black.

3. A well-to-do peasant woman in dark blue bolero and skirt braided in white with the tucked and lace-trimmed white chemise showing as blouse and petticoat. Headkerchief and cummerbund are red and so is the apron which is plaided in black and green. Her stockings are the beige color of Western fashion.

4. A suit of homespun cloth in a gray-brown heather mixture trimmed with dark blue passementerie and embroidery, also dark blue cloth-covered buttons. A garnet-red woolen cummerbund girds his waist. His natural leather carbatines follow the ancient European style laced with leather thongs and the tarboosh is of black sheepskin.

5. Here is shown the jube of padded sheepskin with the skin to the outside, the winter coat of most Balkan peoples. The sleeves are very long with sewn-in sheepskin mittens. The cloak is appliquéd with red cloth pieces, silk-embroidered. The garment folds left to right, held closed by a tied sash. Tunic and breeches are usually white linen, in fact white is a favorite basic color for Balkan dress. A red woolen cummerbund, a black sheepskin tarboosh, knitted red socks and sheepskin carbatines complete the picturesque attire.

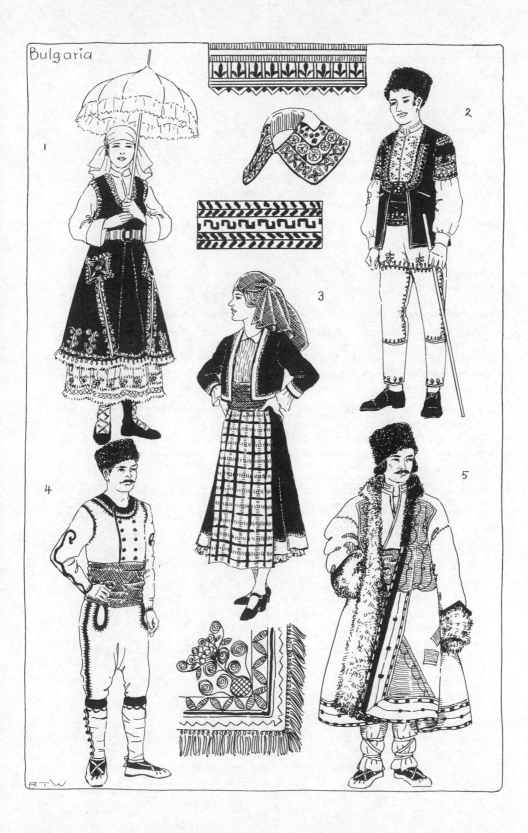

Bulgaria

❧ *Burma* ❧

Plate 31

Burma was formerly inhabited by a people of Mongolian and Tibetan origin. In the 3rd century A.D. Hindus who settled along the coast and at the mouths of rivers converted the Burmese to Hinduism. Then came traders from Europe, Portuguese, Dutch and English. The modern state was founded in the 18th century. Conflicts with the British and government changes followed with Burma finally becoming a Crown Colony in 1937. It was overrun in World War II by the Japanese. By a pact signed with Great Britain in 1947 Burma became independent and a republic.

1. The sarong-like skirt or longyi is worn by men and women. The "acheik" longyi of hand-loomed cloth or silk with a broken pattern of various motifs which most Burmese cannot afford, takes months to weave. The traditional manner of wearing the piece of cloth is wrapping it around the bosom, tying the ends and letting the piece hang. In the illustration it is worn skirt-fashion tied round the waist with a deep pleat to the left of the front, a draping which gives the look of trousers. A white cotton shift is at once blouse and petticoat. The longyi is of striped rose silk with a deep maroon border. Two hats are worn, a straw shade hat with a pink band over a pink cotton turban.

2. A young man in the general Burmese dress in simple white cotton jacket and the sarong-like skirt wrapped round the waist, drawn up to the front left side and tied. The latter may be of cotton or silk and is, in this case, a rich plaid of peacock blue and green crossbarred in heavy black. The black cap is crossbarred in red and the pack-bag is dark blue with red and white ornamentation.

3. A young man in holiday dress. Turban, jacket and breeches are of dark blue cotton or silk with trimming of a lighter blue on collar, sleeves and edge of the jacket and the square on his chest covered with ball buttons. All the buttons, brooches and turban decoration are of solid silver. Chinese shoes of fabric, a red cloth pack-bag embroidered in blue, and a black silk umbrella, the handle, length and fabric of which must follow governmental regulation according to which sex carries the umbrella.

4. Here, the longyi is brought up over the bosom and tied so that the pleat falls to the left side. It is turquoise blue with motifs in rose and white sewn with pearly paillettes. The white organdie jacket is stiffly starched. The dancer's coiffure is dressed in a pony tail with a tiny fillet and fresh flowers.

5. This outfit on the wife of a chief could be worn without change as a chic Western fashion. All the darks in the illustration are deep blue, the upper half of the skirt striped red and gray on a brick red ground. The decorative bands are brick red and blue with turquoise and red accents.

Heads—A very tall and stiffened cap of black cotton or cloth.
A cap fashioned of strings of tiny white and red and porcelain beads. White buttons around the crown and brass buttons dangling from the edge of the cap.
A dark blue turban, the folds accented with narrow folds of red and light blue cloth.
Beaded pendants hang over the shoulder with a silver hoop round the neck.

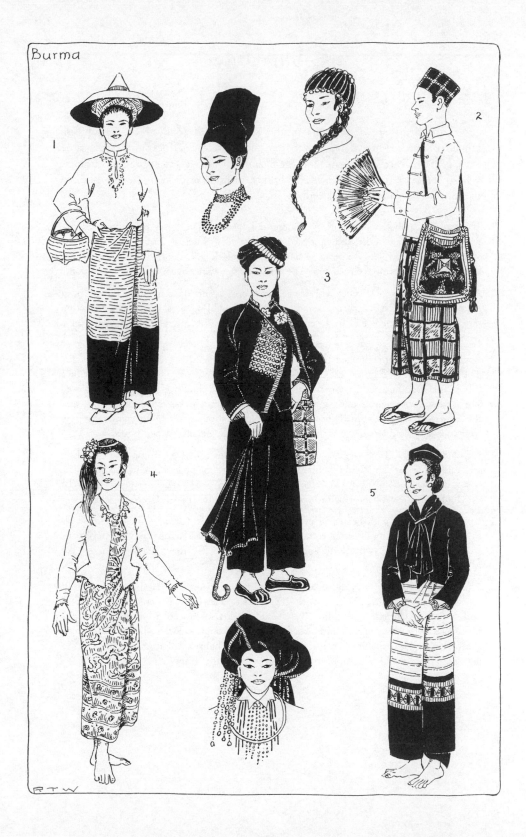

Burma

1

2

3

4

5

✺ Cambodia ✺

Plate 32

The Cambodians are descendants of the Khmers and followers of Hinduism. Cambodia reached its height as a power from the 9th to the 12th centuries. It became alternately a province of Annam and Siam and in 1863, a protectorate of France. It was given more self-government by France after World War II and granted recognition as an independent kingdom in 1955.

1. The typical Cambodian dress of overblouse and sampot. The latter is a length of silk wrapped round the waist, drawn up in front between the legs and giving the effect of trousers. The favored sampot is of dark blue or black silk, the desire for color being fulfilled in a brilliantly colored top. The lady's bag is white with red ornamentation.

2. A little girl of the royal court with shorn head, only a tuft on center top having been permitted to grow. It has been covered with a small gold bowl. To mark the transition into womanhood there will be a ceremonial cutting of the tuft and the growing of a whole head of hair.

3. A girl of the state-maintained ballet school of Pnom Penh, the capital of Cambodia. The sampot of her costume is of heavy metallic silk, shining in gold and silver with a belt of the same fastened by a coral-studded buckle. The shoulder scarf of coral-colored silk is sewn with jewels and embroidery. Necklace and brooches are also coral and the crown is of copper-tinted metal. Gold anklets, bracelets and gold chains hanging from the left shoulder to the right hip are part of formal dress. See figure 6.

4. An official of the Cambodian court in gala dress. The cut of his tunic and his black socks and shoes are in Western fashion. With the tunic of polka-dotted pink cotton he wears the sampot in heavy pale blue satin plaided in black. The red cloak brocaded in white is further enhanced with brocaded bands of white silk.

5. A Buddhist monk with head and eyebrows shaven, in his saffron yellow cotton robe. His wardrobe consists of three cotton robes, two pairs of sandals and one umbrella. Accessories comprise two offertory bags and two fans, one for everyday and one for royal processions.

6. The wedding gown of a fashionable woman of Pnom Penh. The sampot is of metallic brocade in gray, blue and green with a gold belt. The front panel is silver brocade with a fold of Chinese green silk. The shoulder scarf of brocaded copper-colored silk is bordered with silvery green and a ruching of plain copper-colored silk. As in figure 3, she wears the gold shoulder chains, also a diamond chain of intricate design. The bejeweled, embroidered half slippers are simply soles with vamps.

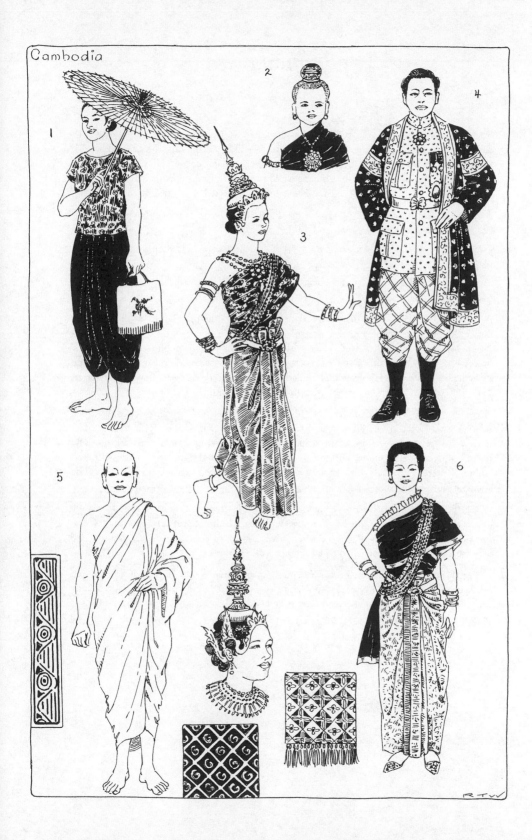

Cambodia

❦ *Canada* ❦

Plate 33

1. Strictly speaking, the scarlet tunic of the Canadian Royal Mounted Police is not folk costume but the dress of the "Mounties" with its silver buttons has become so world-famed as a national symbol that we include it here. Black collar and shoulder marks and black cloth breeches with brilliant yellow stripes. Brown leather belts, holster, cartridge case and field boots and the beige felt campaign hat banded with leather.

2. A member of the Brigade of Guards of the Parliament Buildings in Ottawa in his tall, bearskin cap with white pompon and scarlet tunic.

3. A member of the Royal Canadian Police Guard stationed at the Parliament Buildings in Ottawa, wearing a muskrat cap and a shaggy buffalo coat with leather straps and bronze buttons. Blue breeches and black felt boots with gray wool socks turned down over the tops.

4. A young girl performing the sword dance in the Highland Games at Antigonish, Nova Scotia. Hers is the Fraser tartan of red ground plaided with dark green and a fine white line. A black velvet jacket with silver lozenge-shaped buttons and a black velvet tam-o'-shanter with a silver brooch holding a red cockade and black and white panache. She wears a sheer white, ruffled blouse, knitted socks to match the tartan with red ribbon garters and a sporran in black and white.

5. A piper of the Royal Canadian Highland Black Watch Regiment wearing Nova Scotia's own tartan, a sky-blue ground with black plaid crossed with yellow lines. The dark blue jacket has yellow braid stripes on shoulder wings, cuffs and lappets. The lozenge-shaped buttons and buckles are silver. His knitted hose match the kilt, the ribbon garters are red, a dirk in one sock, and the gaiters are of white linen. The shoes are black and his dark blue bonnet topped with a red pompon.

6. A Caribou Eskimo, native of Yellowknife in the Northwest Territory. His dark blue cloth parka is bordered with beige and red, the fur lining (probably dog fur) showing below hem and cuffs. The breeches, which appear to be a new Arctic fashion, are a combination of cloth and boots of fur with rubber soles.

7. A pretty Scotch bonnet seen in Nova Scotia during gala Week. It is of heather green felt with a puggree band of green and white checked silk. The underband and cockade are of solid green silk with a handsome silver Scotch brooch and a peculiar plume, or perhaps heather.

Canada

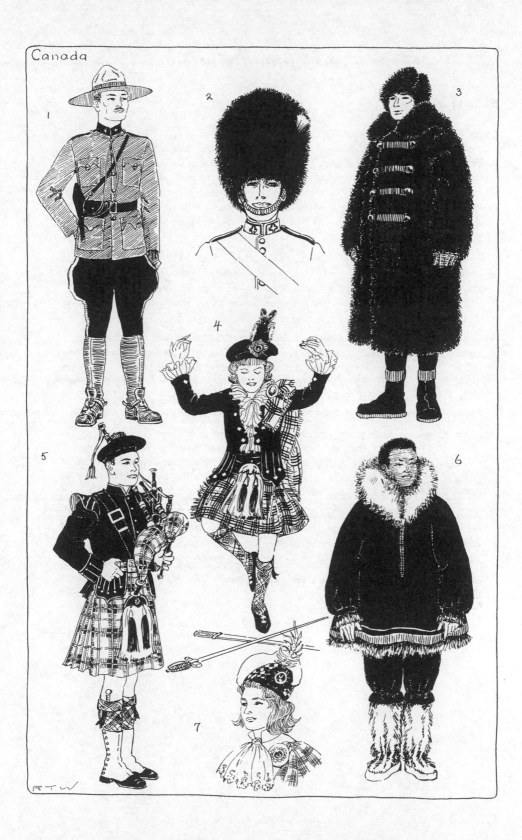

❧ *Canada* ❧

Plate 34

1. An Acadian woman of Nova Scotia in the 18th century dress of her forebears. Acadia, meaning "land of plenty," was the original name of Nova Scotia. In 1755 during the French and Indian War between France and England and their Indian allies many French inhabitants were deported and sent to other English colonies in America. Following the settlement by many Scottish Highlanders it became Nova Scotia in 1784. The costume shown is of white lawn with a black silk apron. The mob cap is also of lingerie fabric finished with lace and embroidery. The lady wears a crucifix of black onyx and her silver-buckled shoes are of black leather.

2. A farm woman of the Gaspé Peninsula in Quebec in the dress prevalent in the late 19th and the early 20th centuries. The frock is of printed cotton, green on white with a capelet of dark blue cloth lined with the print. The apron is striped dark blue, red and pale yellow with which is worn a white lingerie cap, white stockings and black slippers.

3. In Canada the European customs and dress are retained by many groups of foreign extraction. This Ukrainian-Canadian girl of Alberta wears a costume of white linen self-fringed and embroidered in fine stitchery, of course, done by herself. The colors are black, red, orange and yellow. Her black hair is plaited in two braids. Her head-dress is a wreath of red, yellow and white silk roses with gray and white ribbon lappets. The sleeveless jacket and leather boots are black.

4. A young woman of Saguenay Parish in Quebec wearing Saguenay colors on a gala occasion. "Green for forests, red for faith, silver for industry and yellow for agriculture." White are the straw bonnet, blouse and skirt; bodice and upper skirt band of green velvet, narrow bands red, and lowest band, yellow. The bonnet ribbons are of intermingled colors and slippers white.

5. A small boy of Northwest Territory in a red cloth parka lined and trimmed with fur and banded with white and dark yellow cloth. Dark blue breeches and red-topped white skin boots with the fur to the inside.

6. The mother of the youngster in the preceding description in a quilted fur-lined parka of pale blue cotton printed with a pink flower motif. Dark blue breeches and boots like those of the little fellow above.

Canada

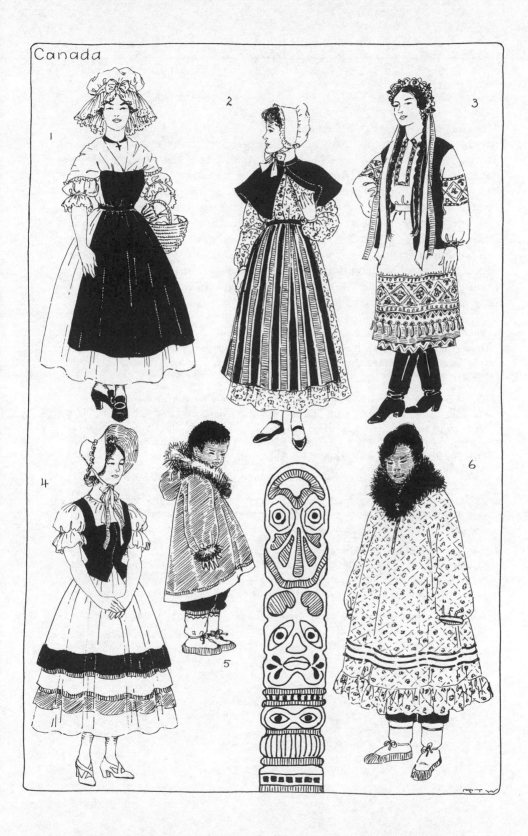

❧ *Canada* ☙

Plate 35   see PENNSYLVANIA (103)

Between 1800 and 1810, Kitchener, Ontario, was settled by Amish immigrants from Lancaster County in Pennsylvania, the descendants today making up more than half of the Canadian city's people. The Amish are a sect of the Christian Mennonites and mostly of German descent. Until recently, Amish people made practically everything they wore except their footwear. The women were always expert seamstresses and even wove the summer hats for summer wear but the black felt broad brims were manufactured by a few professionals. Though their clothes are of drab color and much black, barns and houses are gayly painted red with white trim and the interiors are bright with color. The women of the house occasionally dye a bolt of yardage in cotton or wool in a deep hue of wine red, muted purple or rich blue. And as long as the bolt lasts, it will be used for the mens' and boys' shirts, the daughters' and mothers' dresses.

1. An Amish farmer of Kitchener in his black homespun woolen jacket, waistcoat and trousers all fastened with hooks and eyes. The gray-blue shirt is most likely a "store" shirt because it is equipped with buttons. Black felt hat, gray knitted socks and black leather oxfords.

2. The dress of a farm woman of Quebec City in the last quarter of the 19th century. Of white cotton crossbarred with red, and red bands on sleeves and skirt. A sapphire blue cotton apron striped with white, red and a pale shade of blue. Around the neck, a red cotton kerchief. The white cotton bonnet has a full back and a starched frill. Her slippers are black with white cotton stockings.

3. An Amish woman of Kitchener, Ontario, in drab black with self-fringed shawl.

4. A young woman of Winnipeg, Manitoba, wearing a Hudson's Bay blanket-coat of wool fleece, white with black stripes, yellow round the waist, red next and on the hood and green at the neck. White leather belt and boots, and striped woolen skirt.

5. A French Canadian of Quebec sporting a crocheted cap, white with violet, and a hand-woven sash of red, white and violet wool dyed with natural colors. The decorative, wide sash, a comfortable piece, was popular in the 18th century. Known as the fléchée, the weaving of it has been revived by the Provincial Government today.

6. An Amish schoolboy in black denim overalls and a colored shirt in gray or blue. The hat, shoes and socks are black.

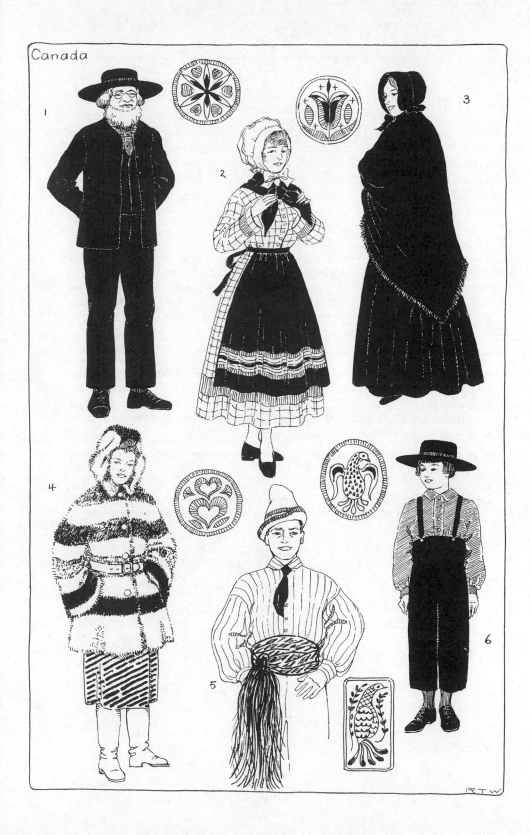

Canada

❧ *Canary Islands* ❧

Plate 36

The ancient name of the Canary Islands was the Fortunate Isles, so-called by the Romans. Peopled by a tribe, the Guanches, little or nothing is known of them except that theirs was a Stone Age culture and that they became extinct in the 16th century. The Portuguese rediscovered the islands in 1341 but a Papal Bull of 1344 gave the Canaries to Castile. The islands were taken possession of in 1402 and have been Spanish ever since.

1. The elaborate dress is but a foil for exquisite handiwork. Of white linen are the blouse, piccadills and tiny apron stitched in fine drawnwork. Also enhanced with drawnwork is the pale green "bunched-up" overskirt. The underskirt of deep yellow homespun cloth is ornamented with an appliquéd black geometric pattern handed down by the early Spanish conquerors who copied the motifs from Guanche designs. A little flat hat of black velvet is worn over a yellow wimple.

2. A sombrero either of black felt or light straw with a ribbon band is worn over a white linen wimple. 18th century.

3. A shepherd in his festival dress in honor of Corpus Christi. Black cloth jacket and pantaloons, the jacket edged with red. A plain white linen shirt and pantaloons, the pantaloons bordered with an embroidered green and a red stripe. The handsome sash is of changeable silk in yellow, orange and brown stripes and white linen gaiters are worn over buff-colored shoes of undressed leather.

4. A miniature model of the costume in number 1 with white linen bodice and apron, the apron stitched in beautiful drawnwork. Of dark green homespun cloth is the underskirt embroidered with geometric designs of red, light green and white. The saucy headdress consists of a black velvet toque with pompons yellow and green, mounted on a yellow headkerchief.

5. A festival costume of white linen shirt and pantaloons with black silk fringed sash and a red or black cloth bolero. A black felt hat with ribbon brides or bonnet strings. White, hand-knitted woolen gaiters are worn with buff-colored, undressed leather shoes.

6. A peasant's hat of the early 19th century of black felt worn over a white linen wimple.

7. A peasant costume with laced corselet and underskirt of homespun cloth with a pinned-up overskirt of striped cotton. The blouse and apron are of white lawn with white embroidery. A tiny white straw hat with wide ribbon band and a huge pompon perched upon a tied headkerchief.

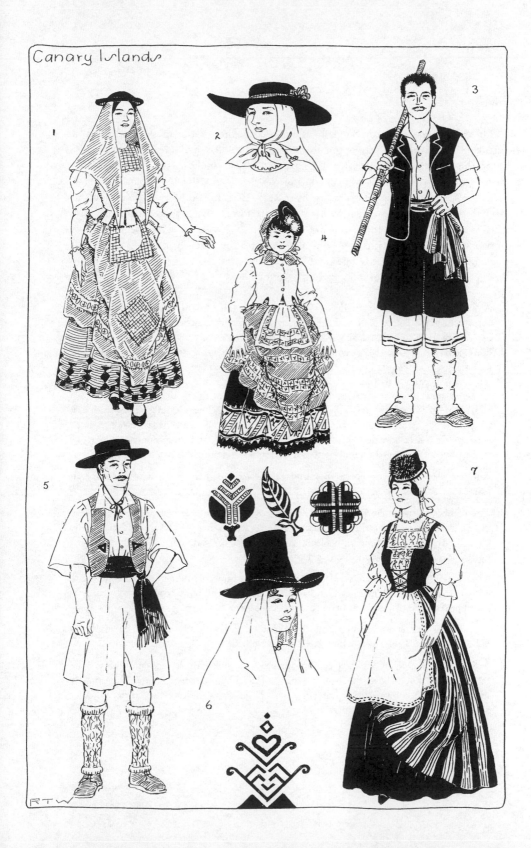

Canary Islands

1

2

3

4

5

6

7

RTW

❧ *Ceylon* ❧

Plate 37

The Island of Ceylon or Singhala is supposedly one of the most beautiful and fertile in the world. It was originally settled by Veddas and Singhalese. In 1505 came the Portuguese, in 1568 the Dutch and in 1796, the English. In 1933, it became a crown colony, was bombed during World War II by the Japanese and in 1948, was granted dominion status by Great Britain. Buddhism, Brahmanism, Mohammedism and Christianity have their followers with more than half the natives being Catholic. Judaism came directly from Jerusalem with the merchants and jewelers. Despite its having been abolished by the English, a caste system still prevails. The Singhalese costume reveals the Indian influence in style and especially in the beautiful fabrics of silks and fine cottons.

1. A Kandy chieftain in the traditional dress of his class. All of silk except the white cotton shirt, the bolero is of dark green woven with the pomegranate motif. The skirt or comboy is of wine color and white over frilled pantaloons of white cotton or linen. This costume of the 1880's remains the same today but footgear has been added in colorfully embroidered slippers and white socks. The comboy worn by all males and females is a part of the national dress. On a man it is wrapped round the figure and gathered above the belt in front. The width and length of the cloth indicates a person's class. One of the lowest class may not have his or hers below the knee. The headpiece of quilted silk is also a sign of nobility. Both sexes and all classes wear jewelry, rings, earrings, bracelets and necklaces and if going on a visit, it is commonly the practice to borrow not only in the family but from friends to complete a display.

2. Another view of the headpiece on number 1, a kind of béret with a tricorne-shaped brim.

3. The comboy as worn by a woman. The skirt and piece over her shoulder are of two different silks woven together, one plain white and the other white with a design. The blouse part is peacock blue with black, and the belt, rose-colored. The hair is dressed tightly into a roll and worn to one side of the head.

4. A page boy in the governor's palace. An all-silk costume of hunter's green and white with a fringed sash. Underneath, he wears a garment of white cotton or linen. His hat appears to be of gilded straw with a gilt ornament.

5. A bridal costume composed of a beautifully draped sari, a family heirloom in mulberry red and ivory, over a sheer, white, laced batiste blouse.

6. A Singhalese noble in a cotton comboy printed in dull greens, reds and ivory. The folds which show above the belt are part of a white undergarment. The smartly shaped flat-topped hat is black but our research does not indicate the fabric, whether felt, straw or cloth over a frame.

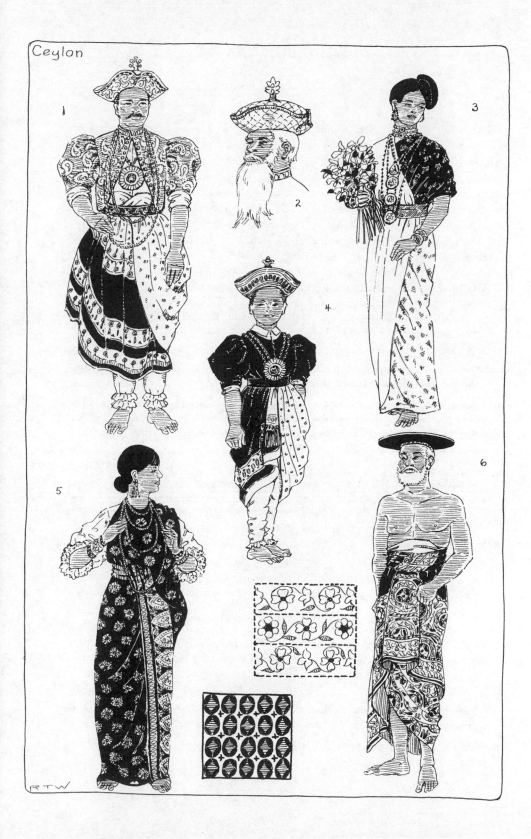

Ceylon

1

2

3

4

5

6

RTW

❅ *Chile* ❅

Plate 38

The South American Republic of Chile on the Pacific coast reaches from Peru to the southernmost point of the continent. The Araucanian Indians were the original people, once the strongest of all South American Indians. In the 15th century Chile was invaded by the Incas from Peru who failed to subjugate the Araucanians. In 1520, the Portuguese discoverer Magellan was the first European to land in Chile; the first invasion of the Spanish conquerors came in 1535. In 1810 the Chileans revolted against Spain. Disputes with Peru, Bolivia and Argentina followed. The country proclaimed a new constitution in 1925, and disestablished Roman Catholicism as the state religion.

1. A Chilean rancher on horseback wearing the hand-woven woolen poncho and a straw sombrero, heavy leather leggings and roweled spurs. The roweled spurs are not used to rake the horse's flesh but are pressed flatly against the animal's sides. The saddle consists of six or seven layers of felt.

2. A ranchman proud of his hat, the handiwork of a hatter of Colchagua Province in Chile. It is a beige wool felt bound with brown leather and embroidered with a design of horses, men, a dog and some fanciful trees.

3. A hauso or cowboy with a light brown woolen poncho striped with red, and a white silk scarf. Dark blue corduroy breeches, undressed leather leggings in brown accompanied by belt and boots of the same. His hat is a gray felt with a ribbon band of a darker shade.

4. The Araucanians, though unconquered by the Incas, did acquire some Peruvian culture such as weaving and silver work. This woman wears the large silver brooch which is worn by all the women, the tupu of the Incas. Her earrings are silver and silver coins dangle from the tupu and the headpiece. Her "modern" costume consists of a hand-knitted, red woolen top and a hand-loomed dark blue woolen blanket skirt. She wears wooden clogs with leather straps.

5. A Chilean rodeo performer in the traditional flat-topped sombrero, of black or brown felt, and the manta, a short version of the poncho. Of hand-loomed wool, its colors are black, white and yellow with green accents in the conventionalized ivy leaf design.

6. An Araucanian Indian on horseback. Underneath the woolen blanket poncho he wears a shirt and the chirapá or pantaloons of guanaco wool formed by being wrapped round the legs and pulled up under the belt. He wears a black felt hat and appears to have no needs of boots, stirrups or spurs, the felt blanket for saddle and a simple loop for the big toe seemingly adequate.

7. An Indian girl with the silver tupu as in number 4. It fastens her cloak, the ichella, a large square of black woolen cloth fringed at the bottom. Around her headdress of two braids is a double fillet of silver coins with a green ribbon bowknot.

8. Showing the carved wooden stirrup with carved undersole and a wooden clog with rubber upper used as a rainy-day shoe.

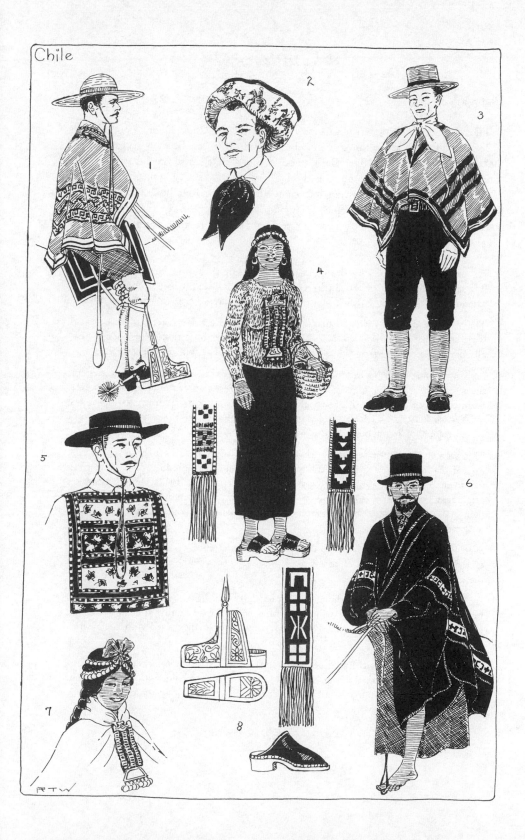

Chile

❧ *China* ❧

Plate 39   see HONG KONG (27), HAWAII (97)

The historic period or written history begins with the Chou Dynasty founded in 1122 B.C. although the Chinese themselves assume their civilization dates back to 3000 B.C. in the Yellow River Basin. The Great Wall against the invasion of the Tartars from the north was built in the late 3rd century B.C. China remained the Chinese Empire until 1912 when it became the Chinese Republic. After years of internal strife the Chinese People's Republic was proclaimed by the Communists in 1949 and the former Nationalist Government moved to the island of Formosa (Taiwan).

1. An extreme version of the cheongsam, popularly known as the Hong Kong sheath. The prescribed length of the slit by Chinese stylists is 8 to 10 inches and should not extend more than 4 or 5 inches above the knee. The dress here is of flowered silk.

2. The working dress for women in the field. Dark blue cotton jacket and breeches. A large shade hat of natural colored straw with deep ruffle of varied color, though usually dark blue, worn over a white headcloth. Wooden clogs with leather straps.

3. Both men and women wear the traditional dark blue cotton jacket and breeches but the man since 1912 has doffed his skullcap for the Western soft felt. He has, however, retained the ankle-length silk robe and the quilted waistcoat, all three garments fastened with buttons and loops. Robe and waistcoat of the well-dressed Chinese are of varied colors but in subdued, artistic, muted tones.

4. This woman in quilted top and dark blue breeches must have been born in the first decade of our century and of wealthy parents, because the binding of a baby girl's feet to shape them into "lily feet" became a penal offense after 1912. The cruel fashion originated in the year 1200 when the Princess Taki was born with club feet. From then on, most upper-class parents would raise one daughter with "little golden lilies" to flatter the princess.

5. So colorful is this quilted cotton costume for a little child that it defies description except to say that the greater part is pink printed with a white flower motif and that the darks are really dark blue.

6. A wonderful turban of a headman in Hainan that would fit into the current Western fashions for women. Of red, white and blue cotton, yards and yards of it wound round, presumably, a brass circlet which is popular in smaller sizes with the women for fillets and earrings.

7. The typical dress of a girl living near Canton. Over her dark blue jacket and breeches, she wears an apron tied in back and held up by a silver chain with brooches. The shade straw hat is mounted on a bandeau and held by a bride tied under the chin.

China

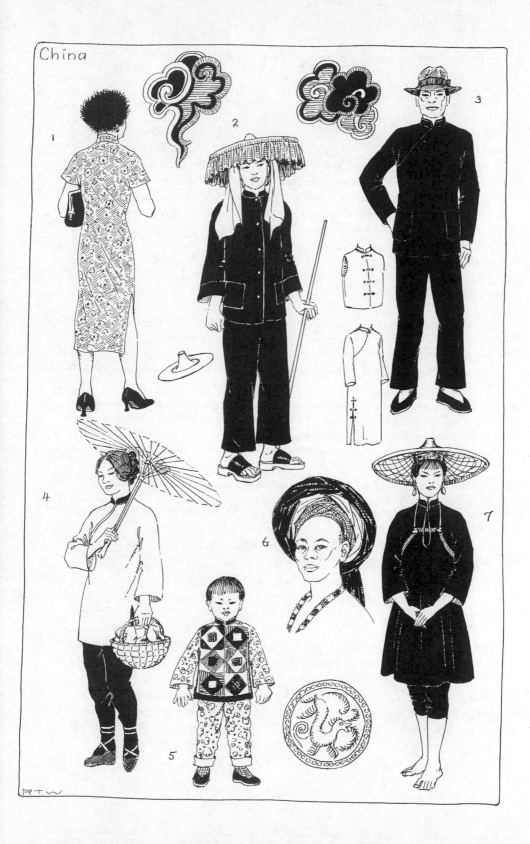

❊ *Czechoslovakia* ❊

Plate 40

During the Middle Ages the Moravian Empire composed of Bohemia, Moravia and Slovakia was overrun 906 A.D. by the Magyars, the dominant people of Hungary. Later, Bohemia and Moravia became part of the Holy Roman Empire. In the 14th century, Prague under the kings of Bohemia was the cultural center of Central Europe. In our century when Austria fell in 1918, Czechoslovakia proclaimed itself a republic formed by the Czechs and Slovaks from territories formerly part of the Austro-Hungarian Empire. It comprised Bohemia, Moravia, Slovakia, Silesia and Carpathian Ruthenia. Hitler in 1939 dissolved Czechoslovakia, making protectorates of Bohemia and Moravia. After World War II, Ruthenia fell to the U.S.S.R. The Republic was taken over by a Communist coup and succumbed to Soviet domination by 1948.

1. A Silesian woman in contemporary dress of moiré taffeta with black corselet and cloak. The bodice is banded with ribbon and worn over an embroidered white cotton blouse. Sash of flowered ribbon with satin edge, held by a gold buckle. White cotton headcloth over a headband of white crochet lace over black. Black silk pantalets and slippers.

2. A Ruthenian miss of the 1870's. Jacket of pelt with brown fur to the inside. Black velvet collar, skirt and picot edging. All stripes are appliquéd red and green cloth. Green wings with appliquéd red stripes. The white cotton blouse is striped in red. Over her hair dressed in a hanging braid, she wears a green toque with red and red velvet streamers. Her boots are of black leather.

3. An elaborately embroidered Slovakian masculine costume. Embroidered ribbons on his black felt hat and forming a cravat of neckband and lappets. The dark blue cloth waistcoat is colorfully embroidered as are the cuffs of the white linen shirt. The embroidery on the dark blue cloth breeches is in gray and black "Austrian knots," done in stitchery instead of military braid. A black leather belt studded with silver nails and black leather boots completes the picture.

4. A Moravian dandy in dark blue cloth bolero and breeches, the bolero enhanced by huge scarlet wool pompons and embroidery. Colored embroidery adorns the white linen shirt. He sports a tiny cap of blue felt or velvet with red cloth crown, and black leather boots.

5. Young Slavic woman wearing a tiara of ribbon and embroidery with bowknot and hanging ends in back. The ribbon is red woven with cut velvet flowers in gray and black and the embroidered band gray and red on white.

6. A Bohemian girl in a black velvet bolero and a black silk apron finely embroidered in white and yellow. A red cloth skirt topped by an embroidered white lawn blouse. The taffeta sash ribbon is woven with a floral design. She wears a red silk headkerchief over a white-frilled cap, her stockings are red and her high-laced shoes are black.

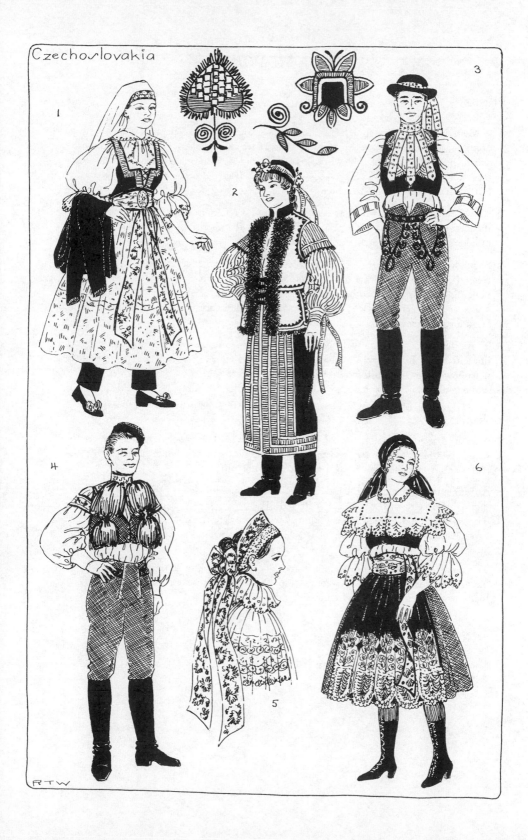

Czechoslovakia

1

3

2

4

6

5

RTW

❧ *Czechoslovakia* ❧

Plate 41

1. A Moravian dressed for church on Sunday. His double-breasted cloak of pelt is edged around the neck with red embroidery. The dark blue bolero is ornamented with scarlet pompons of wool. He wears his hand-loomed, embroidered white linen shirt in loose smock-fashion. The breeches are of blue-dyed buckskin or cloth with black leather boots. The cap of dark blue felt.

2. A diminutive Czech in a blue and white frock with an embroidered pale green blouse, the sleeves tied with ribbons to match. She wears the cherished black silk apron embroidered in white and a pale yellow headkerchief.

3. A Moravian woman with a black corselet having looped edges through which vari-colored ribbon is laced. The black cotton skirt printed with pink roses is sashed with pink ribbon to match. The headdress is a wreath of beaded flowers with ribbon bow-knots and flowers in back. Stockings match the pink accents and accompany high laced leather shoes.

4. These sleeves mark the most distinctive of Slovakian costumes. Of finely pleated white linen or lawn, they are held in shape by being lined with paper. A black velvet bodice is trimmed with beautiful floral ribbon and lace and the skirt is a gayly printed cotton, white and yellow on a red ground. The turban-like headdress is a red scarf with brilliant ribbon stripes. Red stockings match the costume with high laced black leather shoes.

5. A small Czech with fat red wool pompons on his black velvet bolero and red cloth wings with black embroidery and picot edges. He wears roomy, white linen pantaloons and a smart black felt cap topped with a red wool tuft.

6. A Ruthenian wearing a brilliantly embroidered lambskin bolero, the wool pompons in this case being half green and half red. The white smock is colorfully enlivened with stitchery and so are his hand-knitted white woolen socks. The grayish green felt hat is banded with twisted cords of wool in red and green. The breeches appear to be blue-dyed buckskin.

The pointed moccasins worn by the farmer and the small boy above are made of one piece of leather and tied with thongs and, until late years, were the usual everyday footwear for men, women and children.

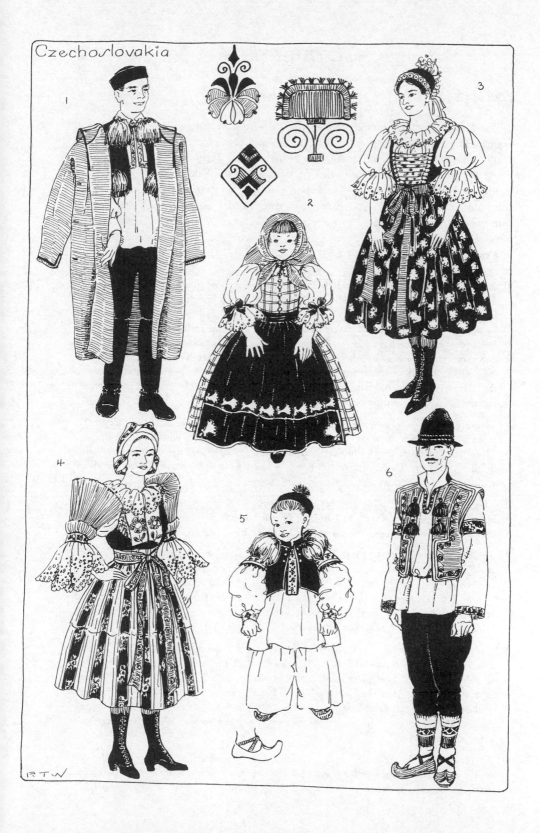

Czechoslovakia

❋ *Denmark* ❋

Plate 42

The Kingdom of Denmark occupies the peninsula of Jutland and surrounding islands. The Faeroe Islands and Greenland are also part of the kingdom. Denmark was settled by the Danes, a Scandinavian branch of the Teutons, in the 6th century. From the 8th to the 10th centuries they participated in the Viking raids on England, France and the Low Countries. In the 11th century they were converted to Christianity under Canute the Great. Next, they came under German influence in the 14th century, being dominated by the Hanseatic League. Today it is a constitutional monarchy. There exists complete religious tolerance but the established religion is Evangelical Lutheran.

1. A Danish noblewoman of the 17th century in a costume showing little change in design from that worn today. The box-pleated skirt and bodice are of hunter's green cloth. The green palatine or cape is embroidered in silk and gold thread and topped by a pleated white lawn ruff. Cuffs and apron are of linen embroidered in white and finished with point lace. Sleeves, leather shoes and pouch are brick red, the shoes decorated with a strip of embroidery. The white felt bonnet is embroidered and the lady carries kid gloves. Suspended by cords to a jeweled girdle are pouch and sheath, the accessory known as chatelaine or housewife because in this manner the woman carried her sewing, knitting and embroidery tools.

2. The Sunday and holiday dress of a man of the Faeroes, a possession of Denmark since 1380. A black cloth suit with knee breeches and a jacket with rows of shining silver buttons. Sometimes the vest is made more festive-looking with colored embroidery. He wears a "liberty cap" striped red and blue or black, black leather shoes with large silver buckles and knitted woolen hose.

3. The bridal dress of a bride and her maids in Fanö. A long white chiffon gown and black velvet jacket with silver buttons. The headdress of flowers and small fruits, perhaps fresh when in season, and a lace handkerchief for good luck.

4. The elaborate costume of the Eskimo woman of Greenland. The tingmiak (blouse) is of silk and skin with a deep collar of fine porcelain beadwork done in brilliant colors. The sekernil (pants) have strips of brightly dyed sealskin in blue, red and yellow. The kamiks (boots) are white skin with the fur to the inside, lace-trimmed and embroidered and worn over the bare feet. Of black sealskin are the standing collar, cuffs and leg bands. The gloves also of black-dyed sealskin.

5. Though this style is also worn by the women of the Faeroes, the bonnet is a distinct feature of Danish costume. Whether of silk or velvet the back is solidly embroidered in colored silk and gold thread and has a bowknot with floating streamers. In green with a picot edge, it is lined with white and has a white frill framing the face with utilitarian green strings tied under the chin. The dress with laced bodice is of plum-colored cloth and the fichu and apron of flower-printed cotton. White stockings and black slippers.

6. These white bushy bearskin pants are called the "trademark of the men of Thule" which is situated at the northernmost end of Greenland. White skin boots, red woolen scarf, a woolen sweater and cap make a dashing outfit.

Denmark

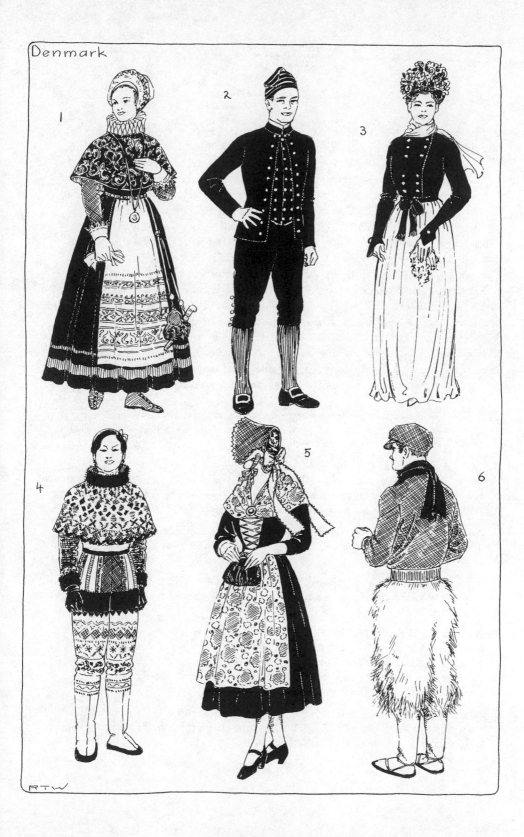

1

2

3

4

5

6

RTW

❧ *Ecuador* ❧

Plate 43

The early history of the Ecuadorian Indians is obscure up to the coming of the Spaniards, their pictographs and writings having been destroyed by the missionaries. The ancient kingdom called Quito was conquered in the 10th century by Indians from the coast. Somewhere around 1500, they succumbed to the Inca armies from Peru. Then came the Spaniards. After three centuries of Spanish rule Ecuador was united to the Great Republic of Colombia in 1822, seceding in 1830 to become a separate republic. The boundaries caused constant friction with Ecuador's neighbors until 1945 when a large section was assigned to Peru. Roman Catholicism is the chief faith. Of the population today, one third is mixed, one third is Indian and the settlement of British and Americans is encouraged.

The Indians of Ecuador are hat-minded people who always wear hats but no shoes. The stiff white felt is the traditional headpiece. It is made of white llama wool and never loses shape because moulded to the consistency of plaster, defying both wind and rain. From Ecuador comes the famous panama hat. Panamas are also made in Peru and Colombia but not in Panama. Though the panama had been made for some three centuries when discovered by the Forty-Niners on their way to California, it became known as a panama because the hat was marketed there.

1. A Quichua Indian in a woolen serape of dark blue, red and white, fringed in blue. A white llama felt hat and a knitted white woolen neck scarf and white linen trousers. The serape opens in front while the poncho has a hole for the head.

2. The rebozo, a pack cloth in which almost anything can be carried. This young Indian woman carries her baby, perhaps lunch and needlework too. She wears her hair in a braid. Her hat is of white felt and so is the baby's. The poncho is red with yellow and black stripes and the trousers are of white linen.

3. An Indian dandy of Otavalo in dark blue and white. The blue poncho is striped with white and the smart looking hat is dark blue felt. Of white linen are the shirt and trousers.

4. A young Indian woman of Riobamba spinning wool into yarn for the weaving of most of the family clothing. Her serape and wrap-around skirt are of homespun in red or dark blue.

5. An Indian girl of Otavalo in an embroidered white linen dress with a dark blue apron, also embroidered. Under the bright blue poncho she wears a mauvish rebozo. The fact that it is not being used and is neatly tied on the left shoulder signifies that she is still unmarried. On her head, the white felt hat, beads around her neck and around her waist a colorfully embroidered woolen sash.

6. A young Indian woman carrying an extra hat, both of felt, one black and the other gray bound with ribbon. She wears her hair in pigtails. The shawl is plum color, plaided in gray and black, the skirt dark green woolen cloth with a black border.

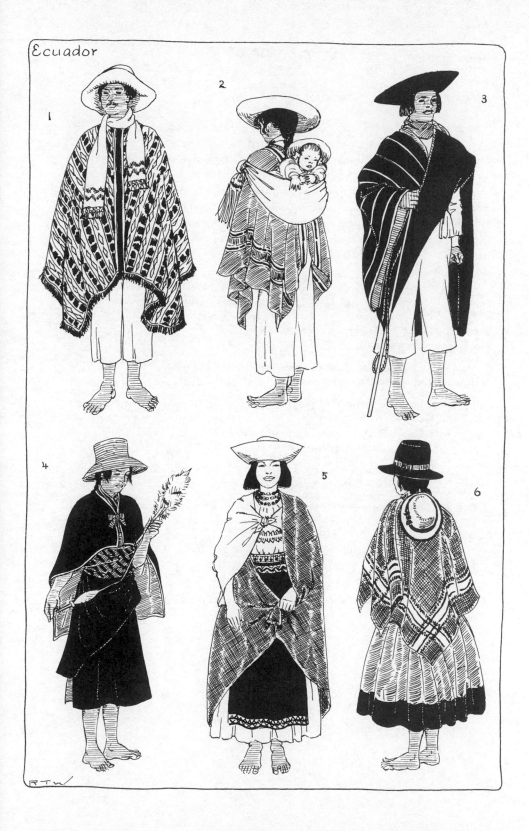

Ecuador

1

2

3

4

5

6

RTW

❧ *Egypt* ❧

Plate 44

Egypt, a republic since 1953, was, as far back as 4,000 B.C., one of the two earliest civilizations of the ancient world. Ruled by native dynasties for centuries she was then part of the Roman Empire from 30 B.C. to the Arab conquest in 640 A.D. Under Khedive Ismail Pasha the Suez Canal was built and completed in 1869. She was declared a British protectorate in 1914 and secured her independence in 1922 and is now part of the United Arab Republic. Egypt is composed of three distinct racial groups—the basic Egyptian Fellahin, the nomadic Arabs or Bedouins and a mixed group, the Nubians. Over 91 per cent of the population is Moslem, a very small per cent Christians and a still smaller per cent, Jews.

1. A man of Port Said in the white muslin costume comprising libas or very full pantaloons, a short jacket with red braid trimming, a double-breasted waistcoat and silk cummerbund, yellow striped with red. The plaited leather cord probably holds his knife. A red fez with dark blue silk tassel and red moroccan slippers with red rosettes complete the dress.

2. A little Moslem girl wearing silver anklets and a checkered tobe. Her hair is cut chrysanthemum style and a ribbon tied round the head puffs the front into fringe.

3. A woman of Port Said wearing a fringed haik of bronze red over her sleeveless black robe. Under that, the tobe or chemise. The yashmak is black with a gold or silver support over the nose and is tied by tapes in back. A white cotton headkerchief covers her hair which is dressed in a hanging braid.

4. A really flattering djellaba and yashmak of fine white lawn with exquisite hand embroidery. Underneath the black haik she wears a long-sleeved tobe of white cotton.

5. A fellah in work dress which consists of libas or pantaloons, a short gandoura of striped cotton and a waistcoat. Over his shoulder he carries an aba and a blanket. The knotted sash might also be a blanket. On his head, the white cotton kaffiyeh and black goat's-hair agal with the ends of the headcloth tied back out of the way.

6. A Moslem woman of Cairo in a black haik cleverly draped "to stay put," the two ends tied on her head. Her tobe is of striped silk. The yashmak with ivory nose piece is of black silk thread crocheted in three different patterns. On her feet, soft yellow leather babouches.

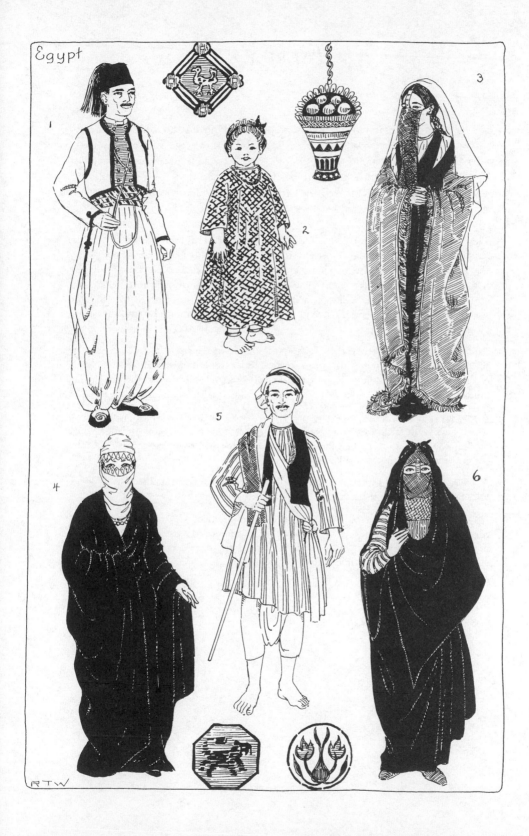

✿ *Estonia* ✿

Plate 45

Estonia is a tiny country occupying a strategic position on the Gulf of Finland. At different periods over seven centuries, it has been under the rule of Denmark, Sweden, the German Knights of the Sword, and Russia. It regained its long-lost independence after World War I but in 1940 Russia again acquired the desired foothold on the Baltic and annexed the little country. Estonia was overrun in 1941, retaken by Russia and annexed to the U.S.S.R.

1. The survival of Estonian national spirit has been aided by periodic folk parades, although their costume today, especially in men's dress, follows a more contemporary trend. This costume consists of blouse and skirt of white cotton, the skirt brilliantly striped. Colored stripes also border the black velvet waistcoat which is belted and buttoned with silver. The flaring tiara is white appliquéd with black motifs. A large silver brooch is worn at the neck and flat black slippers with white stockings complete the ensemble.

2. Among the men, a sports type of dress appears to have replaced the folk costume of yore. This is a tweed suit with knee breeches and silver-buttoned waistcoat of velvet or corduroy. A leather belt with silver buckle, soft shoes of undressed leather and white knitted hose tied with knitted garters of mixed colors make up the accessories.

3. A blouse worn by a group of women in a folk parade in the 1930's. Of hand-loomed white linen with tucked yoke and a fall embroidered in a rose pattern, fancy white stitching and edged with lace. The band of the white-crowned velvet cap is colorfully embroidered and hung with silk ribbon streamers.

4. A sports outfit with pantaloons and checked woolen waistcoat, knitted white wool hose and black leather shoes.

5. A costume of bright colored homespun, the bolero framed with a ruche of yarn of contrasting color. The white lawn blouse frilled at the neck is fastened with the silver brooch which most Estonian women wear. The white-crowned cap sparkles with gay embroidery, stockings are white and the slippers of black leather.

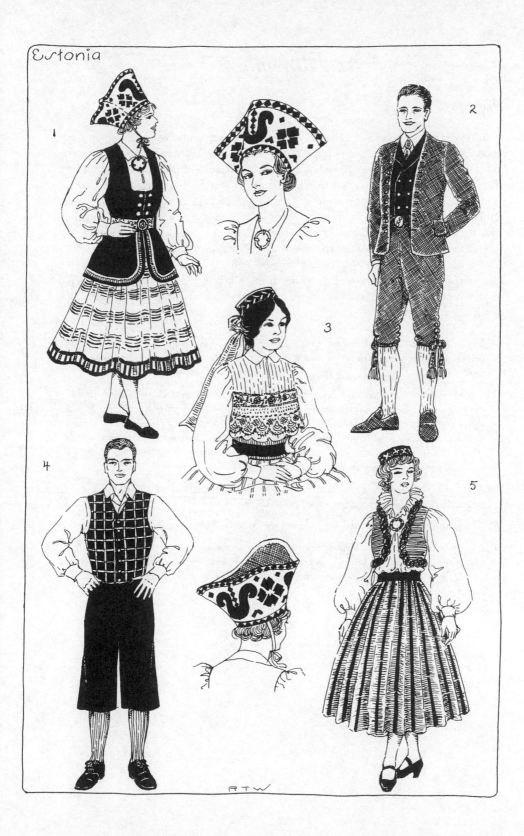

Estonia

1

2

3

4

5

RTW

❧ *Ethiopia* ❧

Plate 46

Ethiopians are a people of Hamitic and Semitic origin and the name Ethiopia is more generally used than Abyssinia. The kingdom has been ruled by a dynasty traditionally descended from King Solomon and the Queen of Sheba and was under Jewish influence until converted to Christianity in the middle of the 4th century. Ties with the Christian world were severed by the Moslem conquest of Egypt and Nubia in the 7th century. With Portuguese aid the Moslem sultan of the Somalis was expelled in 1675. Modern Ethiopia endured various conquests by Italy up to 1941 when she regained her independence after being liberated by the British.

Coptic Christianity is the prevailing religion and the symbolism of the cross is deeply related to the life of the Ethiopians. Every Christian Ethiopian wears a silver cross which is handmade, mostly of silver coin, and which is simple in design and of artistic, native creation.

1. Umbrella bearer to the Emperor in a handsome red cope over a white cotton tunic or wrap-around skirt. Under the tunic is worn the white cotton garment shown on figure 4.

2. A soldier wearing the same undergarment of figure 4 and a wrap-around skirt secured by a leather belt. The Roman toga-like outer piece is a scarf usually of a length of about four yards. The chamma, as it is called, is the principal garment and is worn by men and women with this difference, that the manner of draping leaves the man's right arm free while that of the women leaves the left arm free. Our soldier carries a gun suspended by leather shoulder straps.

3. A young woman carrying a dish of fruit and wearing the gandoura, an utterly simple and artistic robe of cotton or wool belted at the waist.

4. The young man has discarded his chamma the better to pole his raft.

5. A lady in a white cotton chamma bordered with embroidery in deep brilliant colors. Her sleeves denote the same undergarment as number 4 and a skirt, all of white cotton. The long-handled parasol, which is also carried by men, is fashioned of palm leaves.

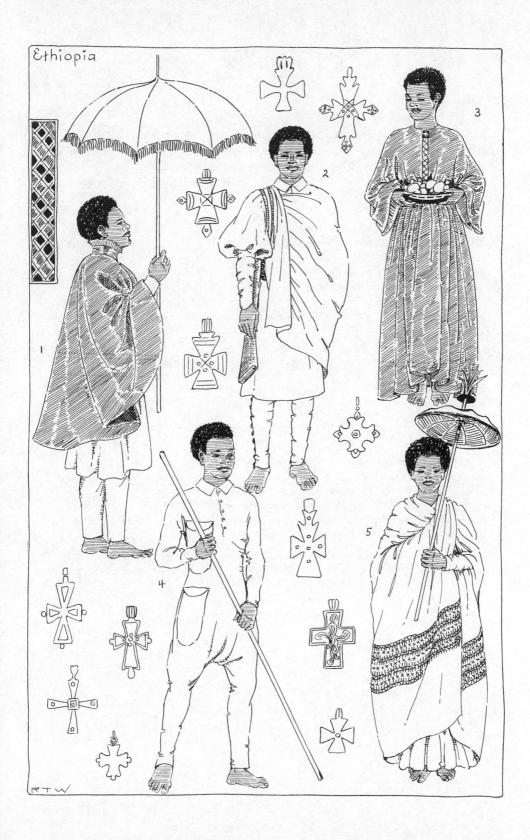

Ethiopia

✻ *Finland* ✻

Plate 47

The original Finns were parts of large Asiatic migrations and of Mongolian stock. In the 12th century they were conquered and converted to Christianity by the Swedes. In 1809 Finland became an autonomous grand duchy of the Russian Empire. A strong national spirit developed and in 1917 Finland declared its independence as a republic.

1. A coat and long, loose breeches of frieze, a kind of off-white woolen felt worn since the 14th century, especially by mountain men. Frieze is a thick, double-woven coat cloth both water- and wind-proofed and finished with a shaggy nap. It is supposed to have originated in the northern Netherlands, Friesland. As shown here, it is usually bound with bright colored cloth, either red or green, often embroidered and fastened with buttons and loops. The hat is of black felt and the footgear, the carbatine, is fashioned of tree bark or undressed leather and gartered with colored cloth ties.

2. A bonnet of brocaded satin ribbon worn outdoors over the frilled white house-cap.

3. A green cloth tunic bordered with white lamb's fur and a heavy silver belt. The white linen blouse and apron are embroidered, the latter bordered with crochet lace. The woman's cap of white lawn has wired wings and her shoes are black leather with white stockings.

4. Over a starched white muslin bonnet with high back and an embroidered frill is draped a silk shawl with embroidered edge and tied under the chin.

5. A Finnish peasant of the early 19th century wearing the favorite apron of black homespun wool embroidered in varied colors, varied stitches and varied motifs. Corselet and skirt are of woolen cloth, the bodice laced with ribbon. The white linen chemise is draped with strings of beads and a silver disk. A ribbon-trimmed turban hides the hair completely and ribbon also decorates the soft shoes of either felt or undressed leather.

6. A jaunty masculine figure in the embroidered, white linen Russian style of tunic and long, full breeches cross-gartered with colored cotton laces. Shoes of tree bark or undressed leather and a black felt hat.

Finland

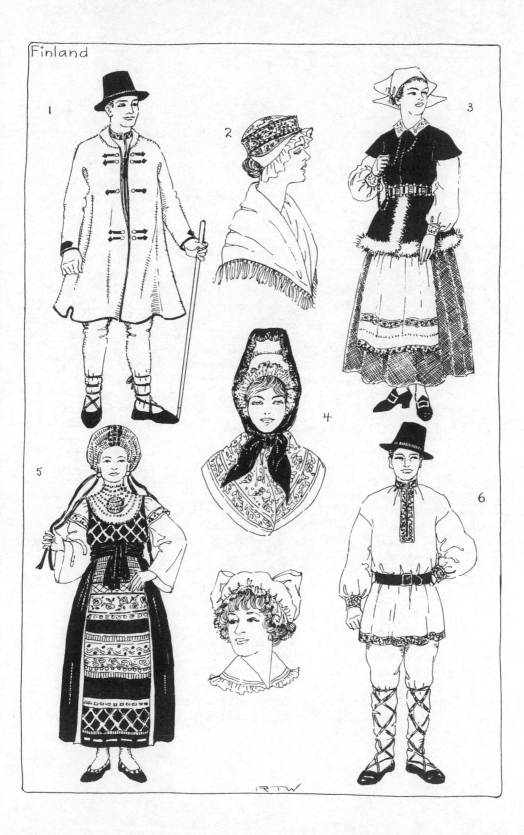

1

2

3

4

5

6

RTW

✻ *France* ✻

Plate 48   see ALSACE-LORRAINE and PYRENEES

France, once a province of the Roman Empire, gradually emerged during the Middle Ages as one of the great powers of Europe under the Valois and Bourbon kings. The French Revolution, 1789–1793, ended the monarchial system, to be followed in the succeeding centuries by republic, empire, monarchy and again, republican forms of government. In 1958, General de Gaulle was elected first president of the Fifth Republic.

Various sections of the country, once separate duchies, retain individual characteristics as evidenced in widely differing costumes, shown here and on Plates noted above.

1. The traditional Brittany costume of double bolero and accordion-pleated breeches, the latter often replaced by trousers full over the hips or by slim trousers. Our illustration portrays a smokey blue cloth bolero with black velvet banding and a black cloth or velvet double-breasted waistcoat with silver buttons. The cummerbund is red, of cloth or silk. The rolling-brimmed black felt hat is banded by a blue ribbon fastened by a silver buckle in back and the ends left hanging. The red-trimmed black cloth gaiters are side-buttoned and worn with either wooden sabots or heavy leather shoes.

2, 3. Two Breton bonnets, both reminiscent of the caps of medieval days, the tall one of the hennin and the pointed one of the escoffion. Both are of starched white lawn with all-white embroidery in shadow stitch and both caps are pinned over starched muslin or buckram shapes.

4. A farmer's wife of Auvergne in a straw bonnet faced with silk and a lingerie frill with a bow at the back. Her dress is of homespun wool and the apron of homespun cotton. The deep cuffs and shawl are of cotton, block-printed in bright colors. On her feet she wears knitted woolen stockings and wooden sabots.

5. A woman of Pas-de-Calais in a fan-shaped cap of lawn or linen and fine lace with bowknots over the ears. With her striped woolen skirt she wears a black bodice and an embroidered fringed shawl. The cotton apron is of solid color. Silver-buckled shoes and white stockings.

6. This woman is a native of Pont l'Abbé, Brittany, a town noted for its embroiderers. The dress is black with embroidered orange stripes for which the town is famous. Over the bodice she wears an orange bolero tucked and embroidered with the unusual feature of lappets wound round the neck to hang in front. The enveloping apron is of lustrous white cotton satin, also tucked and embroidered. The little cap is starched white crochet lace with white lawn ties. Stockings are white and slippers black.

7. Costume of the Province of Berry. The dress is of blue cotton printed in a black pattern and the apron, plain dark blue. With the black cape is worn a coral-colored neckerchief and a large white muslin mob cap.

8. Of Finistère in Brittany, this young man's hat of black felt is dressed with a black ribbon band embroidered with a flower design in white, buckled in back with silver and the streamers hanging.

France

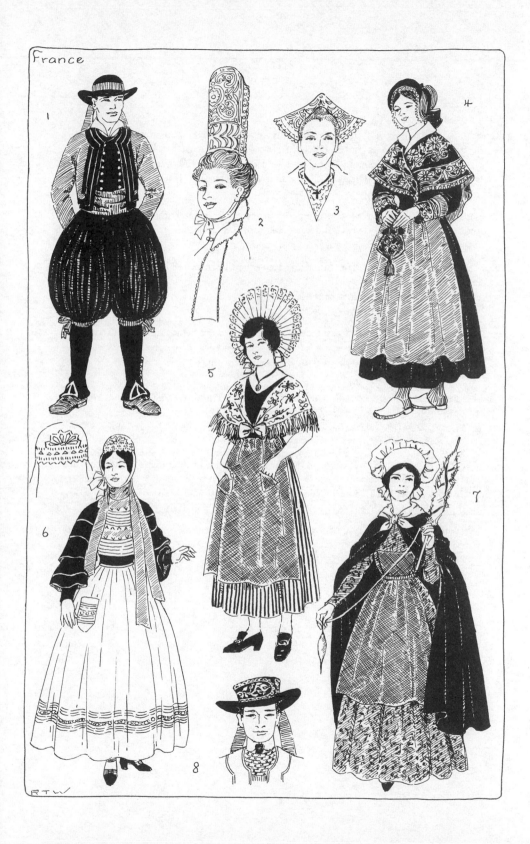

❧ *France* ❧

Plate 49

1. A fête day costume of Finistère in Brittany. A fine color combination for a man is the muted tone of violet and black cloth. Hat, scarf, waistcoat and trousers are black with jacket and cummerbund of violet. The decorative banding near the neck is of a lighter, bluer shade of violet and the buttons are silver. The black hat ribbon hangs in two streamers.

2. A pretty cap of Arles in white organdie embroidered in color with an edging of embroidery. Most generally worn, and very chic too, is the black version, a sort of scarf wrapped round a little cylindrical box of buckram.

3. A Breton costume of Finistère with a tiny lace-edged linen cap. The dress is of woolen cloth with velvet bodice and cuffs. The snow-white lawn collar is finished with a lace edge and the lustrous apron is of cotton satin.

4. A young woman of Bourbonnais in a cloth dress with a velvet border of contrasting color at the hem. Over it, a cashmere shawl and a sheer white apron with the bib and hem edged with crochet lace. Her straw hat is faced and banded with velvet and her silver-buckled shoes are worn with black silk stockings.

5. A farmer's daughter of Normandy in a charming version of the mob cap, a three-frilled cap with a full back, all of flowered organdie. The rest of her costume consists of white linen blouse, striped woolen skirt with rippled braid, a cashmere shawl and a cotton apron of dark color. She wears black stockings with black leather shoes.

6. Breton men embroidered their own jackets. This fête day costume is handsomely embroidered in a solid floral design of several shades of reddish brown, white, and accented with green. The jacket worn over a tailored white linen shirt is of velvet in muted violet and black. The double-breasted, silver-buttoned waistcoat is also violet and black. Hat and ribbon are black and shoes are black in leather and suède.

7. A bewitching bonnet of Normandy in pleated white organdie or fine starched linen with a ribbon bowknot and a brooch.

France

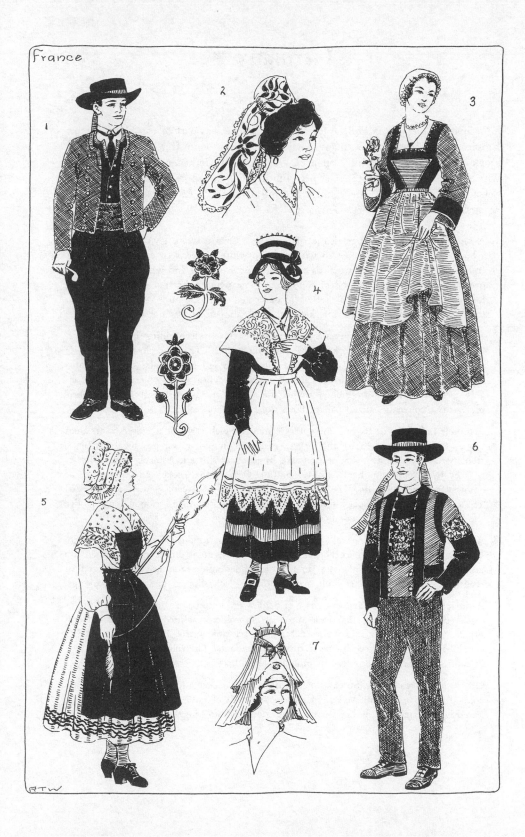

1

2

3

4

5

6

7

RTW

❊ Germany ❊

Plate 50   see TYROL

Germany during the Middle Ages and Renaissance was part of the Holy Roman Empire, being made up of many small principalities and free cities. After the break-up of the Empire by Napoleon, the German Confederation was formed, which eventually became the German Empire dominated by Prussia. Following defeat in World War I, the country became a republic. After World War II it separated into East and West Germany.

1. A woman of Gutach Village in the Black Forest. Over a white lawn blouse is worn a bodice of black velvet embossed with red and white flowers. An embroidered band frames the yoke. The skirt, which is black silk, also has a red and white flower pattern over which hangs a silk apron of solid color. The white straw hat covering a black lace cap, which is for indoor dress, is ornamented with six huge woolen pompons, scarlet for maidens and black for matrons. Black slippers and white stockings.

2. Modern folk dress of East Prussia is composed of black cloth riding breeches, black leather boots and a short jacket of French blue cloth. The red cloth waistcoat is striped with silver gray. The buttons are silver with red buttonholes on jacket and waistcoat. With the white shirt, instead of a scarf, is worn a flat, oblong panel probably secured by an elastic ribbon round the neck. Of silk, the embroidered motif represents a conventionalized pair of birds done in several colors.

3. Feminine folk dress of Bavaria in south Germany, which is given to gayer colors than the northern provinces. Skirt and sleeves of cotton in red, green or blue with black ribbon trim. The upper sleeve sections are smocked or shirred. A black velvet corselet is laced by silver chains held by silver buttons. The bertha, dickey and apron are of embroidered white muslin. The felt hat is either black or green, banded with a cord and ornamented with a black-tipped white feather of down and ribbon loops under the brim. Black leather laced shoes and black stockings.

4. A modern costume of Spreewald that almost defies description. Of embroidered white voile with black velvet bodice and skirt. On the skirt, floral taffeta ribbon edged top and bottom with lace. The floral motifs of bonnet and apron are embroidered in realistic coloring, the bonnet built over padding. Black slippers and white stockings.

5. A modern costume of Föhr, west coast of Schleswig-Holstein province of dark blue or black velvet with a long, full, sheer apron of embroidered white voile. Dark red embroidery below the neck and white ruching at neck and wrists. Pinned on the bodice is a breastplate of silver with fine chains and pendants. The tiara-shaped headdress is of fabric with bead embroidery in muted colors. Black slippers and black stockings.

6. Off to Sunday church in Spreewald in a dark cloth jacket and apron over a brightly colored skirt banded with velvet. Her hood, which is of taffeta, is fairly small if compared with those worn by her friends. The shoes and stockings are black.

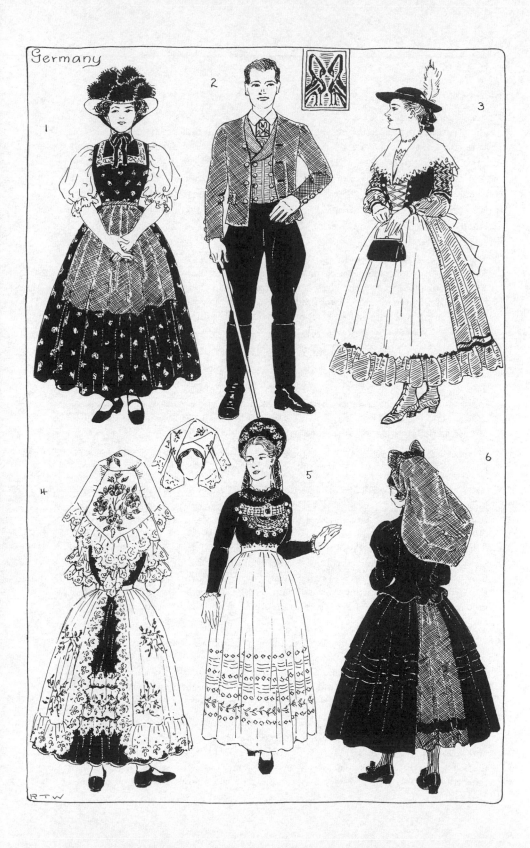

Germany

✳ Greece ✳

Plate 51

The mainland of Greece, the site of early Aegean civilization, was invaded c. 1500 to 1000 B.C. by people of the Balkan Mountains who farmed many small independent city-kingdoms. After its glorious classical period it eventually became part of the Byzantine Empire in the 15th century until its fall in 1455 and was then conquered by the Turks in 1456. The kingdom won independence from the Turks in the early 19th century. Invaded in 1924 by Italy and conquered in 1941 by Germany, it was liberated by Greek and British troops in 1944. The official church is Greek Orthodox.

1. A farmer's daughter near Florina in a black cloth tunic over a white linen chemise. The seams and edging of the black tunic are stitched in red. The front of the waistcoat is silver-buttoned and embroidered in red and yellow and the white chemise is stitched and piped with black. Knee-high leggings of white linen embroidered with red and black wool and a white headscarf.

2. A little lady in Cretan dress and turban of pink taffeta with a corselet of blue-green velvet embroidered in white and fastened by a silver rondel with pendant silver coins.

3. The modern campaign uniform of the evzones of the Royal Greek Army based upon the traditional fustenella in black tunic, black trunks and white wool stockings. A red cap with black silk tassels and red badges and leather belt and cartridge cases. Red tasseled garters and black leather shoes with red or blue pompons.

4. Shepherds and royal guardsmen wear these sturdy, leather, peak-toed shoes or tsaruchia bought in Athens, tufted with red or blue wool pompons.

5. An evzone is a Greek Highland soldier of light infantry who wears the short, pleated kilt or fustenella. This evzone is a Dodecanese. Some 2000 years ago the kilt and bagpipe were carried to Scotland by a mountain warrior of Agricola's army and since, Greeks and Scotsmen have each maintained their own version of the skirl and fling. This shirt and fustenella are of white cotton or linen. The bolero of brown cloth decorated with bronze-colored cording has slashed sleeves, a 17th century fashion. The brown cloth Phrygian cap is weighted down with a brown tassel. Brown leather shoes, white woolen stockings, brown cloth leggings striped with bronze braid and gartered in French blue with matching tassels. The blue is repeated in a striped blue and white sash.

6. A very young Greek in Cretan dress revealing centuries of Turkish influence in its design as, for instance, the fulness of the breeches from front to back. Dark blue waistcoat and breeches with a tailored white linen shirt. Knitted white woolen stockings with shoes having red uppers and blue lower section, a light brown binding and a blue pompon. His knitted cap and fringed sash are vermilion.

7. A young woman of Rhodes in the Dodecanese group of islands in a tunic of black cotton or cloth worn over a white linen chemise. This latter is embroidered in scarlet and yellow, the tunic in scarlet striped with red and white braid. Low shoes of undressed leather in chamois color over which she wears black leather leggings which is said to be a survival of necessary protection against the many snakes in olden times.

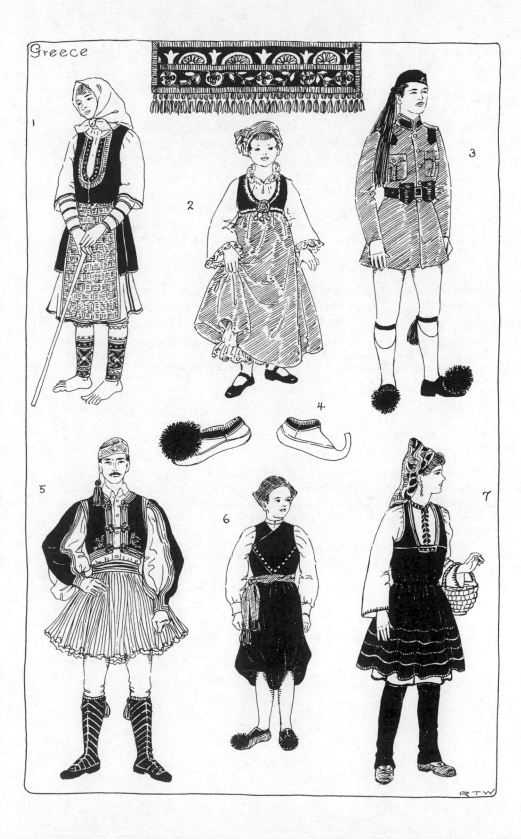

Greece

Greece

Plate 52

1. A mountain shepherd of Epirus in his pastoral dress of dark blue cloth tunic buttoned to one side with a piped blue edging and self-colored sash. Blue cloth cap. White wool stockings with blue garters and black leather shoes with dark blue pompons.

2. A distinctive costume of the village of Trikeri in yellow, black and orange. A sheer yellow chemise embroidered in orange. The apron, also distinctive, is formed of a square scarf or, as here, a square fringed shawl folded diagonally, of yellow or pink. A wide leather belt, fastened by huge gold rondels which are heirlooms, holds the apron in place. A yellow headscarf, white stockings and black sandals.

3. A modern guard wears a uniform based upon this royal dress of the early 19th century, composed of white linen shirt and fustenella with a caftan of blue cloth embroidered in white and a belt of blue embroidery. Red Phrygian cap with black tassel. A red cloth jacket, probably with slashed sleeves, is draped over his shoulders. White wool stockings and knitted blue wool leggings striped with white over black shoes.

4. A rich costume of Epirus in dark blue, gold and rose. The caftan and skirt are elaborately embroidered in gold. A blouse of changeable rose silk. Gold silk turban beaded with pearls and tasseled in blue. Light brown slippers and stockings.

5. A man of Embona on Rhodes in the Dodecanese. His costume is of dark blue cloth with buttoned waistcoat and breeches which are full front to back in Turkish fashion. White linen shirt and neckerchief and a dark blue cap in tam-o'-shanter style with a fur band. His deep sash or "carryall" is of cerise cloth. Black leather boots over bright knitted stockings.

6. The Corfu dress in black cotton, white linen blouse and a yellow gauze apron with orange stripes and lace edge. Milady's bonnet is a flattering headdress of white lawn and lace dressed over a tiara of red roses, perhaps real. The bodice is ornamented with red and yellow embroidery. White stockings and black slippers.

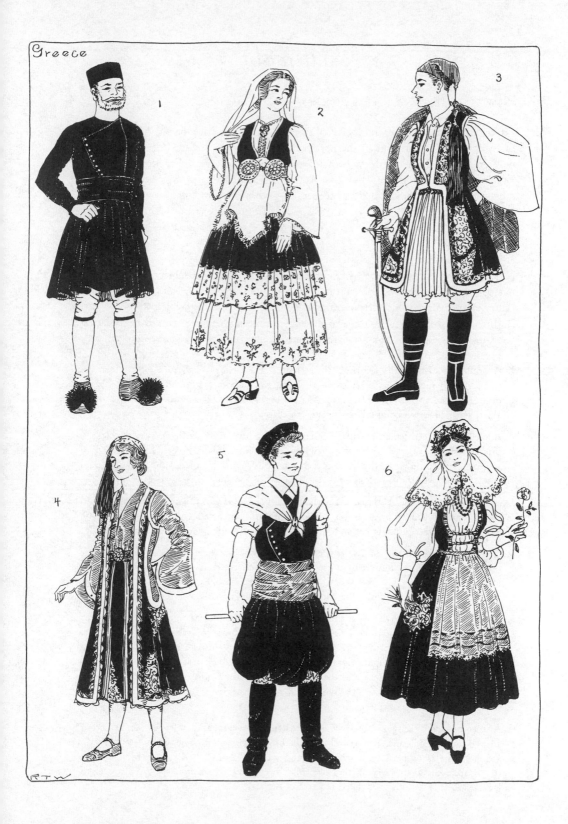

Greece

1

2

3

4

5

6

R.T.W.

❧ *Guatemala* ❧

Plate 53

Guatemala is the most northerly state of Central America below Mexico, with many famous Mayan ruins in the north and ruins of temples and monoliths in the western part. During the first thousand years of the Christian Era the old Mayan Empire flourished on the land that is today Guatemala. It was conquered by Alvarado in 1524 and in 1821, succeeded in revolting from Spain. Guatemala became an independent republic in 1839. The language is Spanish, all creeds are tolerated but Roman Catholicism predominates. Except in the cities, the customs are predominantly Indian.

Practically every piece of cloth worn even today by men, women and children, is hand-woven on home looms of simple sticks. The resulting fabric is therefore of narrow width permitting no cutting, thus prohibiting change of style in dress. Patterns are worked out in conventional designs and coloring which are very gay. Both color and design are unique to the native towns, to change would be violating good taste. The ancient arts of weaving and dyeing survive even in remote villages.

1. A young woman of the Quichés, an ancient Mayan tribe. The tzute which forms a turban but which is also kerchief or servietta, the sash, bag and rebozo (folded) are orange-striped in red and black. The huipil or blouse is black and the wrap-around skirt, dark blue with light blue stripes.

2. A well-dressed gentleman or village elder in a very fine straw hat over a red headcloth. His red shirt is striped in black and white. The white cotton breeches are striped in red, over which he wears the black breechclout. He carries his black and white checked woolen knee-skirt folded along with the fringed black and white woolen blanket.

3. A young woman of Antigua, formerly the capital of Guatemala. Her wrap-around skirt is dark blue and white, a brilliantly colored huipil and a yellowish sash. On her head, what appears to be a white cotton toque is a pad upon which she carries her water jug.

4. A Todos Santos Indian in red striped white cotton breeches protected by the black breechclout which is buttoned to one side. Sash of cotton is striped pink, red and black. A white shirt with red and white collar, a French blue jacket of cotton or wool and a red bandana tied under the hat. Leather and straw sandals.

5. Though colonized by the Spaniards more than four centuries ago, the Mayan race has staunchly held to its own culture. This little headpiece or crown becomes a talisman of the gods, the narrow strip being wrapped round thirteen times and sewn into shape with its Mayan motifs figuring in the thirteens. The colors are pink and sky blue both in the embroidery and the pompons. The huipil and wrap-around skirt are of unusual coloring in sky blue, white and pink. The long gauze scarf is woven in the palest tints of the same colors.

6. A member of a religious brotherhood wearing breeches and shirt of white cotton striped with red, cuffs, collar and sash being of solid red. The knee-length wrap-around skirt is of black and white checked woolen cloth belted at the hipline with the strap used when carrying the skirt folded as shown in number 2. A black cloth jacket and a headcloth of a rolled red cotton servietta.

Guatemala

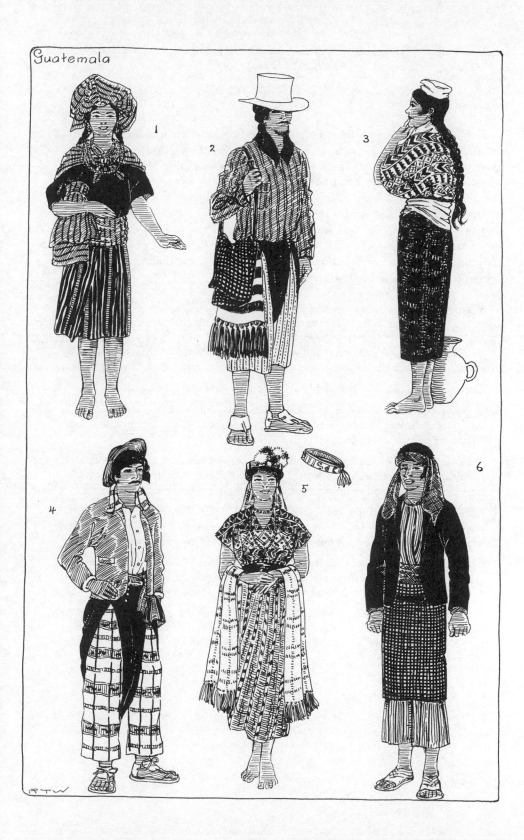

❦ *Gypsies* ❦

Plate 54   see Russia, Spain

A tribe of Caucasian people considered to be originally from India. They first appeared and roamed all over Europe in the early 15th century. No record exists of how or whence they came. Vagabonds and nomadic, they plied their talents as musicians, fortune-tellers and horse-traders in Turkey, Russia, Hungary, Spain and other countries. To the discomfort of the natives many settled in the Baltic forests. Today, their descendants are most numerous in Rumania, Hungary, Russia and the Balkan regions. Their language is considered to be definitely of Hindu origin with some borrowing of words from the lands of their vagabondage. They have neither alphabet nor literature and no religion, in these times generally professing the faith of the adopted country.

1. A gypsy girl in Rumanian costume. The basic dress is checked sky blue and white with a white cotton bolero. The wrap-around skirt is rug-like in weight, made of woolen homespun and gayly embroidered in wools of all colors. The groundwork at the sides is black and dull purple in the front panel and border. A fringed, coral silk headscarf, beige leather belt, shoes and stockings.

2. A felt sombrero, ribbon-bound, and black is the favorite of the male gypsy.

3. A gypsy of Granada in rose and checked cotton sparkling with red satin bands. A small black silk shawl embroidered in varied colors and a flower in her hair. Black slippers and white stockings.

4. A gypsy in Albanian costume. Of white frieze is the undershirt, cummerbund, and pantaloons or chalwar with embroidered suspenders. Frieze is a thick, stout, double-woven cloth of fleece, a favorite among European peasants.

5. Balkan gypsy musician in white frieze pantaloons ornamented with embroidered strips. A waistcoat with braid trimming and a cummerbund of cloth worn over the white linen shirt. A white felt tarboosh, woolen socks and rawhide shoes.

6. A small gypsy girl in Albanian dress. Her pantaloons are of cotton satin, dark blue printed in gray and her blouse, a raspberry-colored cotton with collar and sash in purple. A purple scarf is tied round her head, and she wears rawhide sandals.

7. A gypsy dancer of Granada in a black and white polka dot silk gown with red bands. Checks and polka dots appear to be the favorite prints for the dance dress. She wears the embroidered, fringed silk shawl, a flower in her hair and black slippers with black silk stockings.

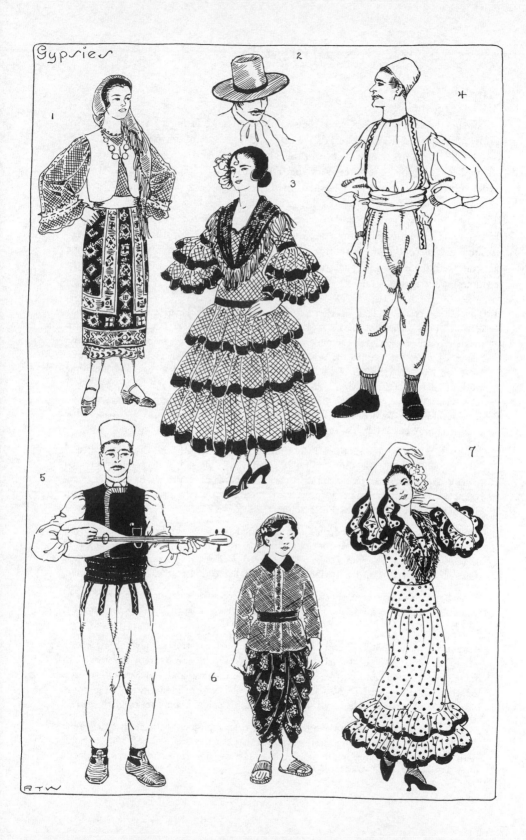

Gypsies

1 2 3 4 5 6 7

ATW

❧ *Hungary* ❧

Plate 55

Though the earliest settlers were Slavic and Germanic, Hungary was overrun by Huns and Magyars in the late 9th century and a kingdom formed in 1001. The country became Christianized early in the 11th century and a constitution was proclaimed in 1222. In the 16th century the Turks took over but were routed by the Hungarians and Austrians. Defeated in 1918 along with the Central Powers, Hungary lost about two thirds of her territory and became a monarchy in 1920. This was dissolved in 1946 and a republic established as the People's Republic of Hungary. The Hungarian language, different from any other European language, is supposed to be the most musical. Under the Communist regime, all religions are tolerated, there being no state religion. The vast central plain makes the country predominantly agricultural.

1. The Hungarian greatcloak or szür is fashioned with wide lapels and a broad sailor collar in back. The enormous sleeves are rarely used as sleeves but are sewn closed, making roomy pockets for carrying possessions. The szür is made of black or white felt or white leather and, in the use of the latter, the fur is worn inside in the winter. Here, we have the cloak in black felt made brilliant with variegated colored appliqué work of cut-out motifs of cloth and leather accented with silk embroidery. The gatyák or wide pantaloons, which look like a divided skirt, are of self-fringed white linen. In some locales the pantaloons are of white woolen cloth bordered with a coarse, white crochet lace. A black felt hat and fine black leather boots with pointed toes.

2. A little boy in the same costume as older unmarried men. A full-skirted gatyák and shirt of white linen. The shirt, embroidered in vivid colors, has sleeves long enough to flare over the fingertips of young bachelors. Young men also wear the gayly embroidered, fringed, black sateen apron. Our youngster wears a green felt fedora with embroidered band and a panache of feathers and flowers.

3. Hungarian cowboys are among the finest horsemen in the world. He wears the gatyák of white linen, self-fringed. Also of white linen is the chemise or shirt with long, full sleeves worn over what appears to be a long-sleeved sweater. A neck scarf, silver-buttoned waistcoat, leather belt and tall, ribbon-bound felt hat complete the dashing ensemble.

4. A cowboy in his cloak of unshorn sheepskin and a green felt hat decorated with a red feather. At night, he sleeps upon the ground rolled up in such a cloak with the hat over his face.

5. A young man in Sunday dress. His white linen shirt has full sleeves trimmed with white lace. The body of the shirt and the black sateen apron are embroidered in orange, green, yellow and purple. The apron in this instance covers black cloth trousers topped by a leather belt. The black velvet waistcoat is ornamented with silver buttons, his green felt hat has a wide, black satin band and his pointed boots are of black leather.

6. A wedding guest in a szür of white felt or leather appliquéd with cloth and leather strips of yellow, green, orange and purple. The pleated pantaloons of white woolen cloth are bordered with a white crochet lace. He wears a turban of green foliage, a silk scarf and his black leather boots sport pointed toes.

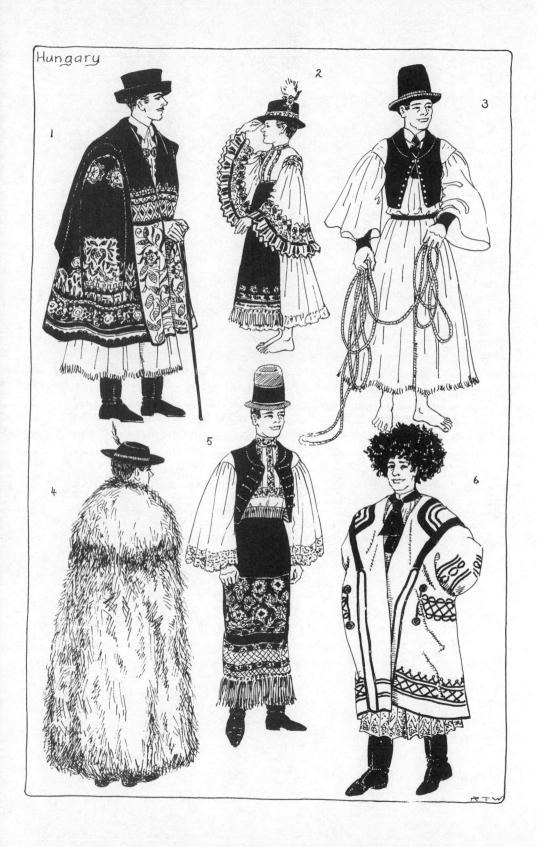

Hungary

❧ *Hungary* ❧

Plate 56

1. A plump maiden in an accordion-pleated, printed cotton skirt over fifteen white muslin petticoats. The white linen apron has accordion-pleated wings, white embroidery, and is threaded with black velvet ribbons. The toque of shirred silk has a rose and streamers of black velvet ribbon. Black leather boots are worn over white cotton stockings.

2. A little girl in her Sunday dress which is a combination of fabrics. Skirt and jacket of printed cotton, the jacket ornamented with black velvet. The pièce de résistance is the black sateen apron just like her elders', colorfully embroidered and finished with deep fringe.

3. A bride in her wedding attire, all white except the bright colored embroidery of the fringed white shoulder shawl. Many strings of beads and chains encircle her neck. The full skirt is pleated and edged with lace. The tiara, worn but this once and called the párta, is a glittering, bespangled headdress of artificial roses in white and delicate shades with floating white streamers in back. On an exquisitely fine handkerchief she carries a candle set in a rose base. Her fine leather boots are probably crimson, that being the coveted color choice in feminine bootwear.

4. A young woman of Alsónyék in a modern version of peasant dress. A lace-trimmed blouse of orange cotton with a skirt of dark brilliant cloth bordered with white embroidery above a black hem. The decorative fillet is a black velvet ribbon with heavy ivory embroidery. The babouches with embroidered uppers are worn with white stockings.

5. A little girl of Tokaj in an embroidered and lace-trimmed dress and a black sateen apron also lace-trimmed. On her head, an embroidered ribbon fillet and on her feet black patent leather babouches and knitted white stockings.

6. The use of color in festival dress runs rampant in all Hungary but the village of Mezököesd surpasses all in its brilliancy. These costumes are often the work of a lifetime and men, during the off-farming season, also take a hand in the needlework. Such garments are handed down from generation to generation. In this case, the skirt is fashioned of printed silk or cotton with black velvet ribbon at the hem. Apron, bodice top and sleeves are of black velvet, the wing puffs of crimson silk and the embroidery in various shades of orange, yellow, green and red. The crimson silk bonnet is heaped high with woolen pompons of crimson and green, and round her neck she wears strings of beads.

7. Black velvet fillet with embroidered motif in heavy ivory silk.

Hungary

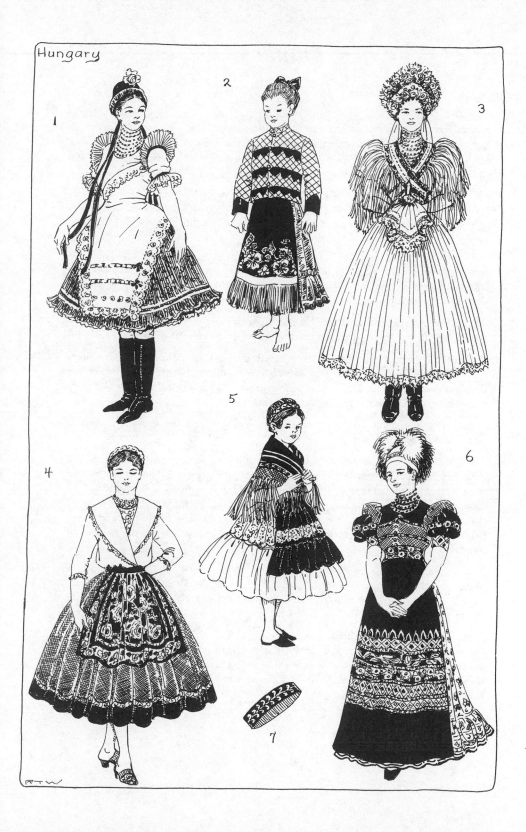

❧ *Hunza* ❧

Plate 57

Hunza, peopled by one of the Aryan tribes of Dardistan, is a protectorate of Pakistan and is a small mountainous kingdom in the Himalayas. It is Asiatic and borders on Afghanistan, Kashmir and China. There exists no written history but traditionally its two thousand inhabitants are descendants of three soldiers of Alexander the Great, who settled there and took Persian wives. The Hunzukuts are fairer of skin and taller than the people of the neighboring countries. Though the people are Moslems, the women, except the ruler's wife who is in purdah, do not wear veils.

1. A young woman in flowing robe and flowing hair. The long-sleeved robe with standing collar and silver buttons is of red challis flowered with yellow. The pillbox is red and draped with a cream-colored cloth. Soft brown leather shoes.

2. A young woman with her hair in braids. A red pillbox with red, yellow and white embroidery and a pea-green chiffon scarf with red, black and white motifs.

3. A Hunzukut guide in coat of red woolen cloth over a brown shirt or smock. Long, full white linen trousers tucked into knee-high boots of soft brown leather which are tied with leather thongs. When on a long trek over the rocky roads, they often carry extra leather to replace a worn sole.

4. A baby boy Hunzukut in a beige cotton garment with half the sleeve of a striped fabric, and a stitched skullcap.

5. The costume worn for the performances of ancient war dances enacted by the men. The dancers wear robes of heavy Chinese silk, some red and some a brilliant dark blue and some of them bordered with brocaded bands of gold and white as in our picture. The robes date from a period when the Chinese emperor paid tribute to Hunza to avoid the attacks along his borders. The robes, curved shields and curved swords are treasured heirlooms of more than three centuries back. Under the robe is worn the costume of number 3.

6. A young man in the same outfit as that worn by his elders. His shirt or smock is orange and the full trousers are dark green. His coat is a woolen cloth of camel's hair color and the heavy shoes appear to be of Western sports style. He acts as servant to the very young relative of the Mir or King.

7. A Hunza girl who has gathered precious twigs for fuel on the barely wooded slopes. Her working dress consists of full cotton trousers striped red and gray on orange which are tucked into the soft leather boots. Next, a red cotton tunic and over that, a dress of tan linen which she has turned up and tucked into her belt. The pillbox is red and her hair hangs in two braids.

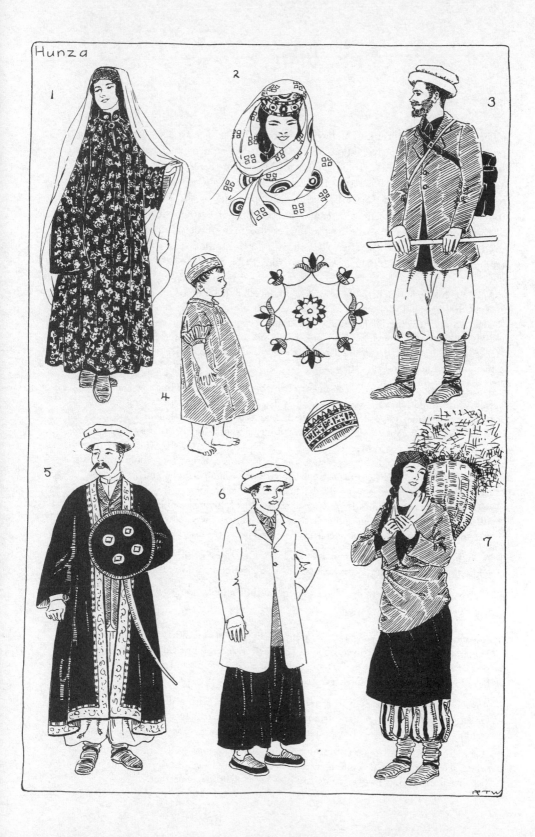

Hunza

❧ *India* ❧

Plate 58

The civilization of the Indus Valley can be traced back at least 3000 years, making India one of the oldest civilizations in the world. Western contact began with the establishment of Portuguese trading posts at the end of the 14th and the beginning of the 15th centuries, followed by the Dutch East India Company. Eventual control over all India was acquired by the British operating as the English East India Company. Civil government was set up and the British Parliament assumed political direction, abolished misrule by the rajahs, also many cruel customs, and spread English education. In 1947 after 40 years of both Hindus' and Moslems' active struggle for freedom, the British withdrew from India as of 1948.

1. An East Indian in modern dress with a high-collared, buttoned-up choga with side vents. It is generally of white linen but may be of fabulous brocade for ceremonial wear. Under it, white linen trousers in jodhpur fashion are usually worn. His turban, called the pagri, is a piece of white or colorful silk or cotton measuring five to twenty-five yards in length. It is wound round the head in various ways, the end either left hanging or knotted on the left side.

2. The sarī is the most important garment of the wardrobe of the Hindu woman or girl from thirteen or fourteen years of age. It is a piece of fabric six yards long and about forty inches wide. Of cotton, silk or both, hand-loomed, embroidered or printed, it makes an artistic costume. The sarī is worn over a short shirt or blouse called a choli of sheer white or contrasting color and a petticoat tied round the waist by a drawstring. The sarī in folds is tucked into the drawstring and wrapped round the waist to form a skirt and carried up in front over the left shoulder. The end is then left to hang or is draped over the head as a hood. Handsome and costly are those woven with gold and silver threads, the metal embroidery giving weight to the drapery. Wealthy women often own a hundred or more and if the need ever arises to sell a sarī, the dealer weighs it for metal content and pays the market price.

3. A Sikh of Ludhiana, considered the world's handsomest men, in a rose silk pagri, white linen shirt, the kūrtā, brown linen or suède jodhpurs and red moroccan slippers.

4. A tarboosh of sheared caracul, shaped like a fez but minus the tassel.

5. The Gandhi cap of white linen.

6. A young Hindu woman of Agra wearing a sarī over a full skirt of red silk brocade bordered with gold and silver ribbon. The sarī is sheer white edged with gold and silver and hand-painted in flowers and pale stripes of carmine and turquoise. A beaded headdress hangs over her forehead.

7. A youthful student of Rajput in a robe of quilted cotton with a diagonally-cut closure. Green cotton printed in red and trimmed with red to match. His draped turban is red cotton striped with black. Over peak-toed slippers he wears brown suède leggings.

8. A Hindu maiden in modern Indian dress of sky blue and rose printed cotton over white slacks. A pale blue chiffon scarf to wear as a veil over her head if she wishes. Her black hair hangs in two braids and her flat sandals are of leather.

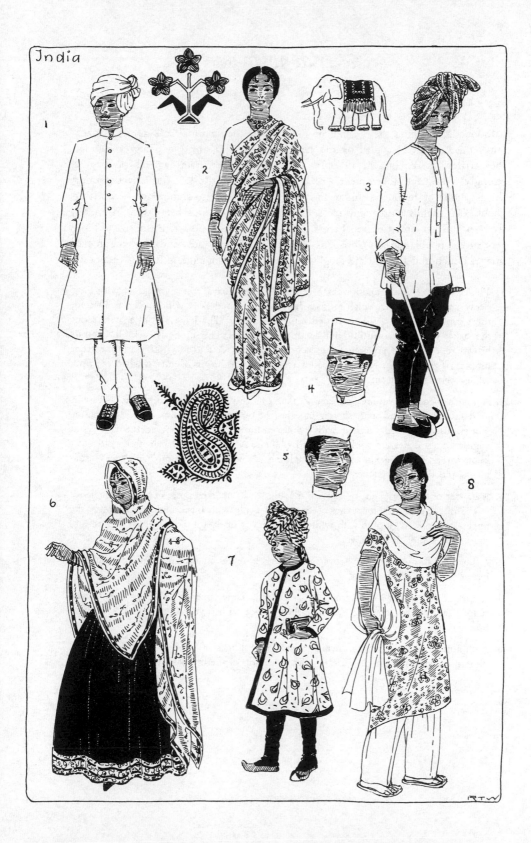

India

❧ *Indonesia* ❧

Plate 59   see BALI

Indonesia, meaning the "Islands of India" was known until 1942 as the Netherlands East Indies. Occupied by the Japanese 1942–1945, the Nationals proclaimed
the territory a republic in 1945. In 1950 the member states agreed to form a
strongly centralized government with an amended constitution, formally becoming
the Republic of Indonesia. Indonesia is the world's largest archipelago comprising
about 3000 islands with many races, the four largest islands being Java, Sumatra,
western Borneo, and Celebes. Bali, Lombok and Timor also rank in size. 10 per
cent of the population are Christians and Hindus, the 90 per cent, Moslem. In language, Dutch and English are taught but the official language is Bahasa Indonesia.

1. The costume of the Javanese woman consists of the kabaya, a straight jacket with long
   sleeves, and the sarong which forms a long wrap-around skirt with a deep front fold,
   the garment held by a silk scarf tied round the waist. The kabaya is often white but
   the jacket shown is nasturtium pink with white motifs. The sarong is dark blue, red or
   brown following the preference for deep-toned colors. A fold of white edges the front
   drapery. Typical of the feminine headdress is the draped cloth of muslin whether in the
   village or working in the field.

2. A man's wedding costume, an heirloom of the 18th century of dark blue silk with
   gold motifs combined with shorter breeches of turquoise blue also with gold motifs.
   The trouser legs are finished with white embroidery. Crossed over the chest and
   edging the breeches are scarlet and gold ribbons. A white leather belt with gold bowknot, carved ivory buckle and sheath holding a kris. Dark blue cap with ivory ornaments and dark blue leather sandals.

3. A dancer of Surakarta, one of a group moving in the stylized poses of an ancient dance
   to the music of a tinkling orchestra. Sarong of beige with black and green motifs, the
   upper section of dark blue with white. The scarf is of deep brilliant green chiffon and
   she wears a tiny silver crown.

4. A Javanese farmer in white cotton shirt, dark blue cotton breeches and the umbrella
   hat or bamboo chapil.

5. A girl of Timor, one of a group of snake-dancers wrapped in a heavy cotton robe
   striped red, yellow and black. Tortoise-shell crown with silver filigree, silver comb and
   bracelets.

6. A Sumatran latex plantation owner in working clothes of white cotton shirt, a pale,
   pleated cotton sarong, a black cloth stylized version of the tarboosh and leather sandals.

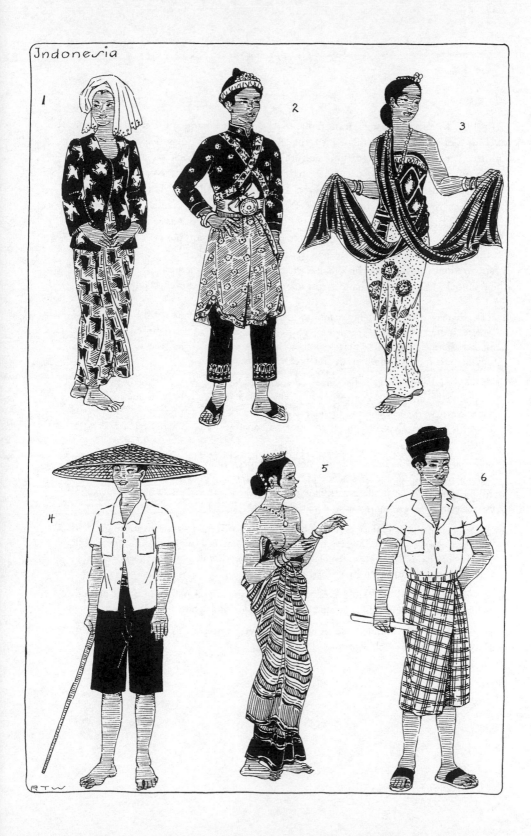

Indonesia

❊ *Iran* ❊

Plate 60

In 1935 by official decree, Iran replaced the ancient name of Persia, a nation of Indo-Germanic people related to the Aryans of India. Based upon Oriental culture, Persia has a military and cultural history dating back to antiquity. She was conquered by the Moslem Arabs in the 7th century and after conquest by the Mongolians in the 15th century, became a Mongolian dynasty. Modern Persia has been ruled by shahs who held off the Turks but lost to the Afghans in the 18th century. In the 19th century the Persians lost territory to the Russians. In the 20th, Persia acquired a constitution and adopted a westernizing policy. The wearing of turbans and fezzes was restricted to government leaders. In religion that of Islam predominates. In the history of art, their miniature painted illustrations and their embellished texts in manuscripts of calligraphy have never been equalled.

1. The chadar, that enveloping mantle which was banned in the 1920's in favor of Western dress, has been revived by women who like it as a comfortable wrap in winter. Formerly all black, now, especially in summer, it is to be seen in light colors, gay flowered prints and often, in all-white over Western dress.

2. A piece of headtire which has come down from the days of the Persian Empire is worn by the men of the vast Kashgai Tribe which is legally subject to the Iranian Government. Of thick felt and in color, light brown, it takes various shapes on various heads. The flaps are worn up at the sides, fore and aft, or down over the ears in winter.

3. A country woman in her working clothes. A sheer cotton frock, pale blue printed with a pink rose design and worn over baggy trousers. These latter, called chalwar, fitting snug at the ankles, are dark blue cotton figured with red and yellow. To conceal her face she wears a cap, mask and veil all attached and of black chiffon.

4. A member of the Bakhtiari clan in a combination native and Western hunting outfit. Checked cloth jacket and white linen shirt are combined with the traditional silk pantaloons, a cloth or lambskin kolah on his head and white canvas shoes. A leather cartridge case is suspended by-crossed straps.

5. A little girl in a printed cotton dress of blue and white floral motifs on a red ground. White collar and cuffs and a knitted bonnet in black and white.

6. A Persian worker in brown woolen cloak and trousers over a bright blue cotton shirt. His hat or kolah is of black lambskin or cloth.

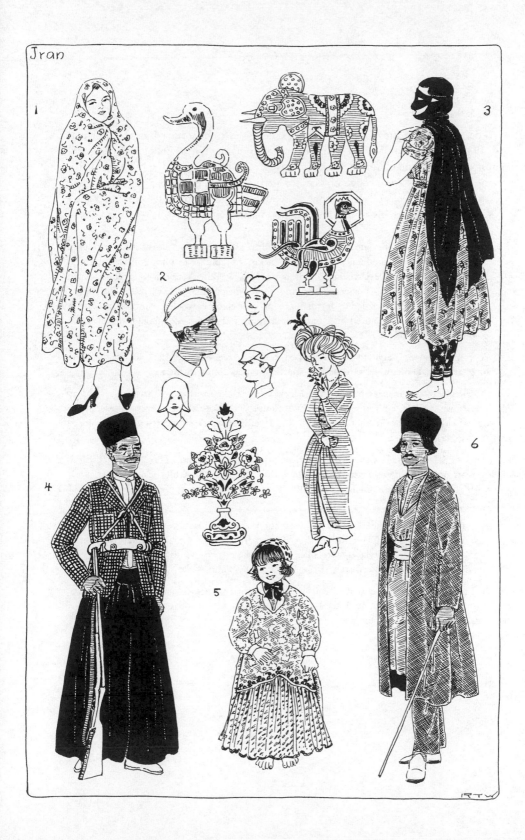

Iran

❧ *Iraq* ❧

Plate 61

The independent kingdom of Iraq was established from former Turkish territory in 1921 after World War I. Iraq, the modern name for Mesopotamia, includes most of Mesopotamia and the Turkish vilayets of Basra, Baghdad and Mosul. It became a member of the League of Nations in 1932 and was occupied by the British to prevent Nazi control. It is now a republic. The people are preponderantly Moslems with Christians numbering about 150,000.

1. A Turkish lady of the late 19th century in an "at-home" costume of rose and gold color. Chalwar or pantaloons, caftan and jacket of gold silk with gold thread embroidery. A wide girdle jeweled according to one's wealth. A smock-like blouse worn with the pantaloons is of sheer white and shows below the jacket cuffs. The calpac or cap and the cloak called a feridgé are of rose-colored woolen cloth. The cap is bound with a richly colored silk handkerchief and the peak-toed boots are of gold-colored suède or velvet.

2. A young man of Baghdad in his striped caftan, a sleeveless jacket, no doubt made of goat's-hair homespun cloth, and a smartly draped cotton turban.

3. A college student in peasant costume. Black velvet jacket with gold thread embroidery worn over a sheer, embroidered, all-white blouse with Dalmatian sleeves. The chalwar of red cloth with woven motifs, a white head veil and black slippers with flesh-colored stockings.

4. Pairs of boatmen pole the long canoes along a canal in Basra. This Arab's costume consists of a striped cotton turban, white cotton shirt and dark blue cloth jacket worn with the skirt-like pantaloons. His dark blue half-socks may be of knitted wool or of leather.

5. A Jewish matron in the early 1920's wearing the loose, black veil or shale with the yashmak of horsehair. Over this she has draped the aba, an Arabian square of fabric, here a light-colored, polka-dotted silk. Under these two wraps one notes the embroidered hem of a Western style dress. Black slippers and white stockings.

6. A Turkish villager in his striped cotton caftan sashed with a colorful silk scarf. White cotton shirt and trousers. Peak-toed shoes of rawhide in natural color and the red fez without tassel.

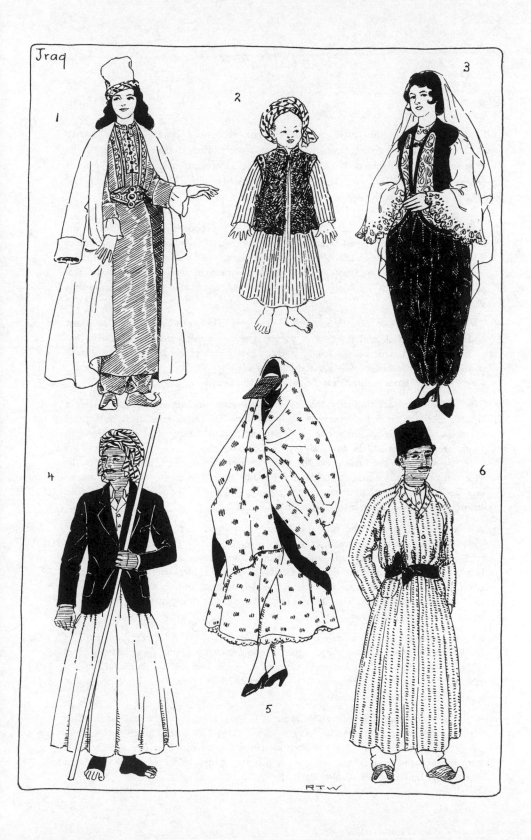

Jraq

1

2

3

4

5

6

RTW

✳ *Italy* ✳

Plate 62   see TYROL

The peninsula of Italy after the fall of the Roman Empire was for many centuries made up of small city states. These were united under a king in 1861. The government was seized by the Fascists under Mussolini in 1922 in the "March on Rome". In 1945 Italy was invaded by the Allies and in the same year the Fascist Government was overthrown. Italy became a republic in 1946.

1. A woman of Sardinia in festival dress with a slashed bodice of green panels embroidered in black and piped with scarlet and worn over a full-shirred white blouse. The underbodice or corselet is white with black border and also piped in scarlet. The black skirt has a dark red border and over it an apron of white polka-dotted black silk. Her headdress is a folded, black fringed shawl, the whole costume reminiscent of the 16th century.

2. The masculine version of number 1. A bolero of scarlet cloth with panels of green embroidered in black and piped with scarlet. The full pleated shirt and breeches are of white linen. A wide belt of felt or leather heavily embroidered holds a black cloth flounce with corded edge. The knitted black woolen cap can be worn in innumerable ways, and necessaries or lunch can be carried in the pocket end.

3. The festival costumes of Sicily are the most elaborate in Europe. Albanian Greeks who accepted the offered sanctuary of Sicily to escape Turkish oppression have retained the dress of five centuries ago, but it is disappearing today because of its costliness in fabric and handwork. The gown shown is red with wide bands of gold lace and a gold fringe around the hem. Over the skirt, an apron of fragile black lace. Over the sheer white blouse, formerly the chemise, the lady wears two quilted capes, the under one black with gold embroidery and the outer one, French blue with silver and gold embroidery. On her head, a tiny cap of red and gold.

4. A villager of Merano in the Alps reveals an Alpine look in his dress. The red cloth jacket and vest are trimmed with two shades of green, a dark tone and a bluish shade with a touch of silver on cuffs and neckband. The buttons are silver and the black belt is enhanced with silver braid and embroidery. The black velvet breeches have silver piping. He wears a white linen shirt under the vest and white hose accompany silver-buckled black shoes. The dashing black felt hat carries a panache of plumage in white, black, red and tawny color.

5. A young woman in Taormina's contemporary festival dress. The vermilion skirt is bordered with sapphire blue with a gold ribbon band above and above that, a silver ribbon. The yellow cotton blouse is threaded at neck and sleeves with black velvet ribbon. The jewel of the costume is a sheer white voile apron with drawnwork and a deep frill of exquisite reticella lace.

6. A young man wearing the festival costume of Foggia based upon the style of the 18th century. The habit is of charcoal gray woolen cloth worn with a cloth waistcoat of black and gray-blue plaid. A white linen shirt and a hat which is a rhapsody in pink, felt, ribbon band and flowers all in the delicate shades. Black shoes with ribbon rosettes and knitted white woolen stockings.

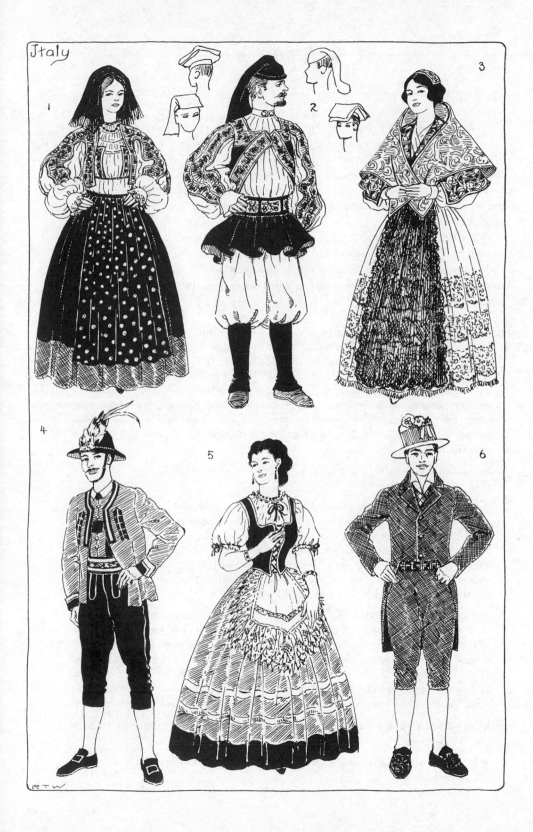

Italy

1   2   3
4   5   6

RTW

❧ *Japan* ❧

Plate 63   see HAWAII (97)

Japanese history dates from 660 B.C. with accession of the ruler of the royal line, Jimmi Tenno. The Portuguese in the 16th century were the first Europeans to visit Japan and in the same century Christianity was introduced. Eventually, contact with the Europeans was cut off by decrees of the rulers. Commodore Perry in 1854 succeeded in obtaining the first commercial treaty which was followed by the adoption of occidental civilization. Buddhism and Shintoism are the principal religions.

The elegant and artistic kimono remains Japan's national costume for men, women and children despite the fact that Western costume is being worn more and more because of its practicality. Men, especially outside the home and when traveling, have adopted Western dress. All garments of both men and women fasten left to right.

1. A geisha or "singing girl" in a black satin cloak or "haori" embroidered or painted in red, white and gold floral pattern. The under kimono and the sash or obi are of vermilion silk embroidered or painted in gold and white. The embroidered collar of the fine white chemise shows above the neckline of kimono and coat. The crest of the wearer is embroidered or painted in center back, on both sides of the chest below the shoulder and on the lower back of the sleeves of both kimonos. She wears white cotton tabi or stockings which are fastened in back with tiny hooks, and felt sandals or zori with ribbon straps. Her lacquered hair is dressed with flowers and sprays of symbolic rice.

2. A little tot wearing an outer and under kimono in light-colored printed cotton tied at the neck with ribbons.

3. A bride in her wedding raiment with a real hat in mauvish-pink chiffon and flowers as the headdress. A kimono of white silk crêpe is the underdress of the magnificent outer kimono. The latter is of silk painted in yellow, orange, red, black and tawny shades. The obi, about fifteen feet long by about a foot wide, is here three stripes sewn together, two of solid red and one figured. The butterfly bow in back puffed with a small cushion is worn only by maidens and brides. The zori are covered with brocade and her tasseled fan is tucked in the obi.

4. The man's kimono is practically the same as the woman's but with shorter sleeves. Over a loincloth of muslin and a silk or cotton shirt, he wears two kimonos, the collar of the under one rolling over the collar of the outer. In formal dress over the inner kimono are worn loose trousers of stiff silk which look like a divided skirt. There are six pleats in front and five in back and each side slit part way down from the belt. The two kimonos and the trousers may be of different colors but all are muted and dark. The black silk coat usually carries the family crest on each side of the chest.

5. A lady in the rain in a waterproof silk cloak of light color; cork or wooden clogs or gēta.

6. A farmer in homespun linen shirt and breeches. Gartered footwear made of rushes, and a straw hat.

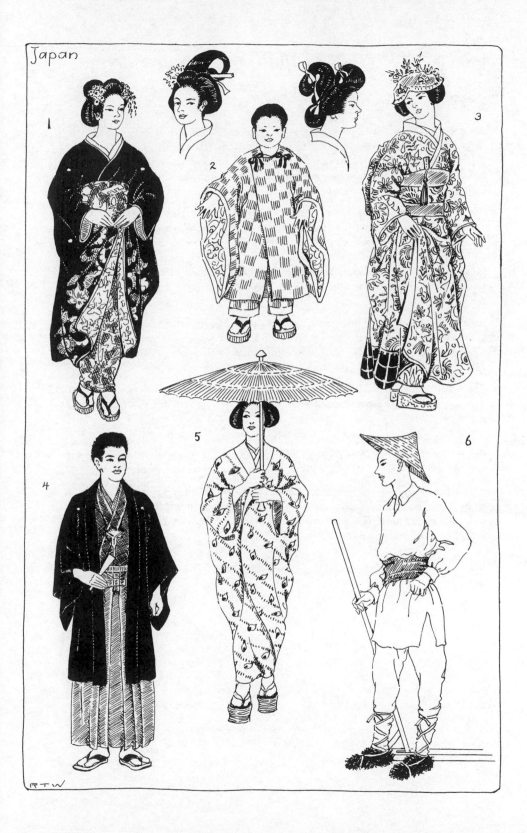

Japan

1

2

3

4

5

6

RTW

❉ *Japan* ❉

Plate 64

1. A maiku or young novice in training to be a geisha. The maiku is designated by the long flowing obi. Maiku dress is governed by various traditional colors whereas the geisha is free to choose color and design. Flowers and sprays of rice ornament her headdress. The white cotton tabi are fastened in back and the clogs have wooden or cork soles.

2. Farm girls when working prefer pants to skirts. The dark blue pantaloons are tied on over a kimono of printed cotton in light blue on a dark blue ground. The pantaloons of this "three-apron-costume" are open at the sides. Red suspenders, a red and white sash and upon her head, a square of white cotton or linen printed with decorative motifs. Hands and arms are protected by black mitts of rubber or plastic fabric; some men also wear such mitts. This young woman wearing zori is engaged in scattering seed.

3. Another farm girl in her three-apron work costume. Her red and white striped cotton breeches are tied round her waist over a cotton kimono, white with gray printed motif. The suspenders and sash are red cotton with a single white stripe on the sash, and the gēta or wooden clogs have blue leather uppers.

4. The fisherman wears a dark blue shirt, gray cotton trousers, straw hat and a raincoat. The waterproofed raincoat of dried grass will be drawn up over his shoulders, should it rain.

5. A young unmarried woman with the obi dressed in back over a small cushion called the obiage. The obi is of pinky-beige stiff silk and the kimono, an apple green silk with marbleized design in white. Her zori are brown with brown ribbons.

6. A member of a group of pilgrims on their way to visit a shrine. They usually dress in white. His short under kimono could be red, dark blue or white. He wears an unusual style of the zori made of leather with heavy soles and laced in front. Straw hat and mitts like those noted in figure 2.

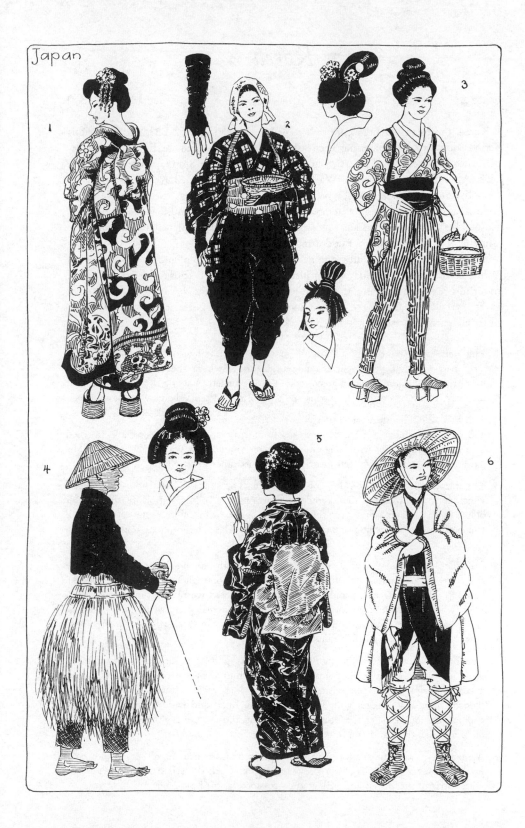

Japan

❋ *Korea* ❋

Plate 65   see HAWAII (97)

Korea, the Hermit Kingdom, has a recorded history since 57 B.C. and at various periods down the centuries has been associated with the Chinese Empire. Its independence was recognized by treaty at the conclusion of the Sino-Japanese War 1894–1895. After the Russo-Japanese War 1904–1905, Japan occupied Korea and in 1910, forcibly annexed Korea as Chosun or "Chosen". In 1945 it was freed from Japanese control and by agreement a temporary line divided the military occupation of Korea, between the Russians and the Americans. The principal religions are Christianity, Confucianism, Buddhism and Chondogyo.

Korean festive and wedding clothes are of silk, which is plentiful and luxurious. White cotton is for every day and principally for adults. Because of long periods of mourning and white being the color of mourning, white became the traditional everyday color. Children are dressed in gay colors. As is the case with the Japanese, all garments fasten left to right.

1. The Keisaing or dancing girl in an all silk costume of yellow taffeta over a red robe. Trimmed with red, yellow, green and purple, the black in the drawing is intended for purple. Red moiré sash and green moiré floating panels. A white silk blouse shows at the neck. Headdress of beads, ribbons and silk tufts, and white boots with peaked toes.

2. A man's wedding attire of scarlet silk overcoat over a white silk "waistcoat shirt", and white pantaloons secured by cords tied round the ankles. The overcoat is fastened by a one-loop bowknot with long ends. A purple ribbon sash with silver buckles. The hat and boots are black, of felt or velvet, the boots piped with white.

3. The traditional white cotton dress of the women. The skirt is pleated to a bosom-band which is snugly fastened round under the armpits. A full-sleeved white silk vest or blouse is put on next and over that goes the bolero with colored embroidery and a one-loop bowknot fastening, the same as the man's. The bolero may be pink or robin's-egg-blue.

4. An older gentleman in white silk coat fastened with the one-loop bowknot, white silk shirt and pantaloons. His hat is woven of black horsehair and worn over a horsehair cap which protects his topknot. Masculine hair was worn in a pigtail until marriage when it was dressed into a topknot. Only married men wear hats, bachelors going hatless. A cone-shaped oiled yellow paper or silk cap carried folded in the waistcoat protects the head when it rains.

5. The bride, who wears white in her daily life, is garbed in brilliant color for her wedding. Over the white silk blouse and the bosom-high skirt of purple silk she wears a coat of bright green silk with an embroidered red silk belt and an embroidered plastron. The long sleeves with white border are lined and banded with red, yellow and purple, the black in the illustration meaning purple. On her head, a tiny crown of beads, silk tufts and embroidery and on her feet, white shoes.

6. A member of a farmer dance team which gives performances in off-season and competes with other teams. The everyday white cotton work dress is made to look festive with scarfs of green, red and yellow and occasionally, bird plumage.

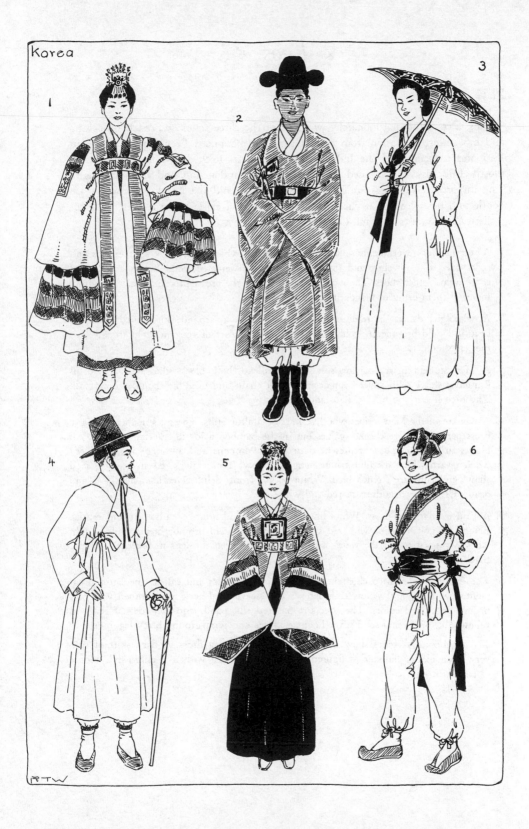

Korea

1   2   3

4   5   6

RTW

✣ *Laos* ✣

Plate 66

Laos, a constitutional monarchy, was one of the three states of French Indochina and has suffered invasion from earliest times. It became a French protectorate in 1895 and a member of the Indo-Chinese Union in 1899. The mixed population, mostly Buddhist, is composed of people of Thai-Indonesian and Chinese origin. The important languages are French and English and the people themselves are gentle and peace-loving. A chaotic, political situation exists today created by Neutralists, Communists and anti-Communist factions.

1. A secretary of governmental office, the members of which wear black silk turbans and coats over a white shirt and trousers. Some go barefooted, some wear sandals and some wear leather shoes. The ivory badge worn on the breast proclaims their standing, many of them being of mandarin rank.

2. A schoolgirl dancer in traditional Laos dress, a wrap-around skirt called sinhs, of beautiful gold brocade. A gold metal belt holds a scarf of red and gold thread over the left shoulder.

3. A Meo student in a "pyjama suit" and skullcap, both black silk, with a colorful knitted sash. A solid silver hoop-necklace and chain and over his shoulder a carryall. The Meo live in the hills of Laos and Vietnam.

4. A woman of the Man Tribes who live in the Tonkin Hills. The girls in their barbaric dress perform in live checker games out in the bamboo fields to entertain visitors. All blacks in the illustration represent dark blue. Pompons and apron of fringe of red woolen yarn with dark blue fringe hanging below. Trouser legs red and white. Tied shawl and cuffs are French blue. White bodice front. Solid silver hoop-necklaces and beads. Crownless headdress of red and white silk.

5. A prince in formal dress. White linen coat with gold brocade cuffs, belt and marks. Baldric of gold brocade with red stripe. Sampot of gold brocade, a piece of straight fabric wrapped round the waist and drawn up between the legs in breeches fashion. Black leather boots.

6. The daughter of a Meo chieftain in a black velvet dress and calpac, the latter ornamented with red and yellow embroidery. The sleeves and neck are trimmed with silk printed in muted colors. The overskirt has red silk bands and a border of red and yellow silk. She wears solid silver hoop-necklaces and wrap-around black leggings.

The thumbnail sketches show Laos women in marketing dress. A dark skirt of silk, very often black, plain or of figured silk which is worn with a Western-style blouse of cotton in light color.

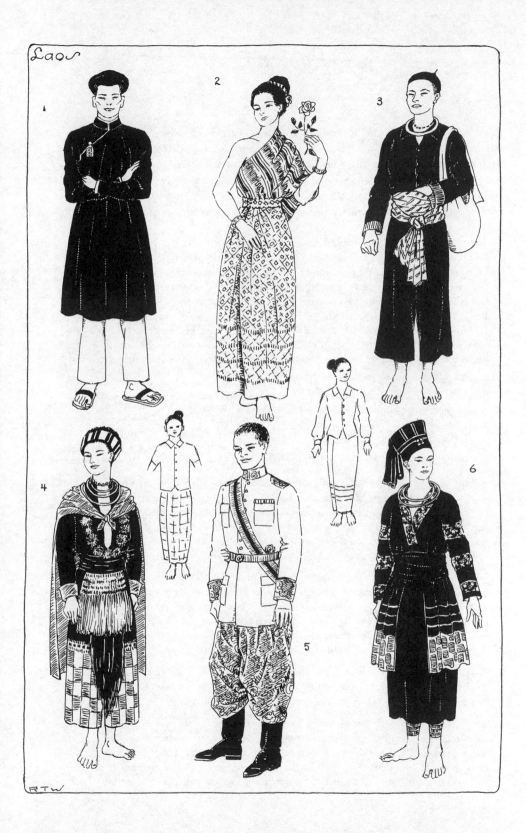

Laos

❈ *Lapland* ❈

Plate 67

Two thirds of Lapland lie within the Arctic Circle, spreading south into the northern parts of Norway, Sweden, Finland and Russia. Being neither a geographical nor political entity, the Lapps have always suffered subjection by the countries mentioned, although more consideration than formerly has been shown them since the 19th century. All that is known about them is that they are a nomadic, Mongolian race, formerly being constantly pushed farther into the north.

1. The favorite colors of Lapland dress are dark blue with scarlet trim but this outfit worn by an older man is brown with red. The long tunic, called the kapta, and breeches are of reindeer-skin for winter and of cloth for summer wear. When reindeer skin is used for dress and some other purposes, the skins are dehaired as well as tanned. In severe weather two kaptor are worn, the under one with fur next to the body. The "hat of the four winds" or "sorcerer's cap" has given way to a peaked cap. Of this cap, brown with red piping, the wearer said that he used the cap outdoors as a pillow, three points being stuffed with down. The fourth point served as his purse. His peaked, leather shoes, mutukas, are stuffed with reindeer moss or sedge grass.

2. A very gay knitted cap in scarlet with yellow and dark green pattern and a wide black band. A picturesque tassel of reindeer strips dyed brilliantly in the same colors. His tunic is of rare and expensive white reindeer piped with red cloth.

3. Gradually, folk dress is being replaced by Western clothes as young men migrate to the cities. Here, one sees the traditional blue cloth tunic with red and yellow embroidery, but the blue cloth breeches are of jodhpur fashion and the leather shoes Western style.

4. A little girl in a reindeer-skin coat with collar and cuffs of red cloth embroidered in yellow and belted with a braided thong belt. Her fur boots, probably dogskin, have reindeer-skin soles with the fur to the inside and are stuffed with sedge grass. Over the reindeer-skin breeches she wears brightly colored wool socks. Her bonnet, of traditional design for women and girls, is of scarlet woolen cloth embroidered in yellow and perhaps a touch of dark green.

5. Women's dress of dark blue cloth with cuffs and skirt border of red striped with yellow. A red apron banded with yellow and a wide yellow belt with red and blue embroidery. The implement dangling from the belt is a knife or pukko which is carried by some women and by all men. The red bonnet has red and yellow embroidery and a white lingerie frill around the face. The breeches are dark gray bound with anklets of red wool and the peaked shoes are of reindeer-skin.

6. A little man in his dark blue kapta and breeches elaborated with red cloth and fancy stitchery. The cap is blue embroidered in red and yellow and topped with the masculine pompon of red wool. A braided leather thong belt and rubber "store boots."

7. The contemporary folk costume of the male Laplander. Tunic and breeches of blue-dyed reindeer-skin, the tunic ornamented with red and narrower yellow stripes. He wears a wide, strapped leather belt from which is suspended his knife. Around his body is the lariat of braided deerskin thong rubbed well with fat to keep it flexible. Blue peaked cap with red band and pompon, red anklets and peaked reindeer shoes.

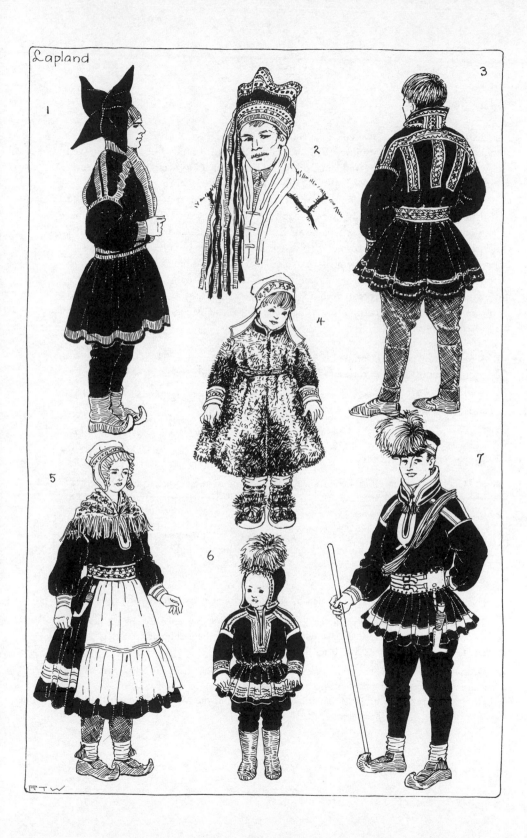

Lapland

❋ *Malaysia* ❋

Plate 68   see SINGAPORE (27)

Off the southern Malay Peninsula, Sumatra, Central Java and East Borneo were colonized from the 1st century B.C. by Hindus from India. This was followed down the centuries by the influence of Buddhism, then Confucianism in the early 15th century and Mohammedanism in the 16th century. In turn came domination by the Portuguese, the Dutch and the British in modern times. Seminaries and institutions of higher learning were established by missionaries and the principal religions are Christianity, Confucianism, Buddhism and Chondogya. In September 1964 the Federation of the former British territories was to become a new sovereign nation in southeast Asia in which the colonial areas of Malaya, Singapore, North Borneo, Sarawak and Brunei would unite under the name of Malaya. Brunei withdrew and as of 1965, forces within and without appear to be planning an expansionist policy by incorporating Singapore with the Malay Peninsula forming a "Greater Indonesia".

1. A farmer of Malacca in printed cotton shirt, sarong and turban. The sarong is yellow with red motifs and the shirt and turban are dark blue and white.

2. A little boy in white cotton shirt and trousers with a silk sarong plaided in dark blue and wine color.

3. A little girl in a deep sky blue silk jacket and sarong, the jacket edged with white embroidery and fastened with pearl buttons. Her hair is dressed in a topknot and her sandals are brown.

4. A Malay woman of Singapore in an all-silk costume. The sarong is plum color with shadowy gold pattern and her wrap of white damask is brocaded in gold thread. On her feet are brown sandals.

5. A Chinese girl of Singapore wearing the cheongsam or "Shanghai dress" of brocaded silk damask. It is not considered proper to wear the slit higher than ten or eleven inches.

6. A Malay woman of Perupok in an orange shawl, a bright blue jacket printed with black and white flowers accompanied by the silk sarong in two shades of brown.

7. This Malay and the boy in number 2 wear their sarong shortened by rolling it up at the waistline. It is dark green silk with white cotton or linen shirt and trousers. Black felt tarboosh, black socks and black leather sandals.

Open-top pillbox hats that were a favorite of Sarawak women in the early part of our century. Colored bead embroidery on silk.
Fringed collarettes in brightly colored cotton thread that the Malay women of Sarawak spin, dye and weave themselves.

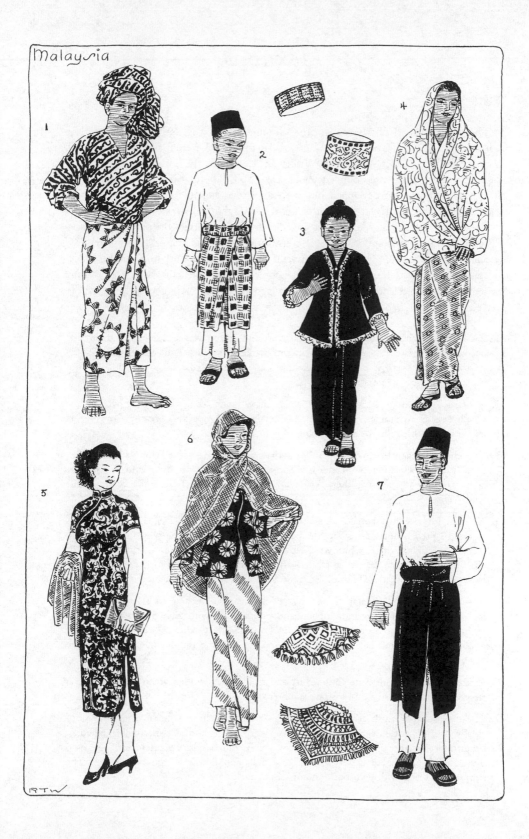

Malaysia

❊ Mexico ❊

Plate 69

The vast tableland of Mexico in pre-Columbian days was the home of a highly advanced Indian culture. The Mayans built pyramids of heroic size and invented a calendar. The Aztecs reached the Valley of Mexico in the 14th century and the capital, Tenochtitlan, was founded about 1325 A.D. The culture of their predecessors was absorbed and developed but with an added horrible cruelty. Cortez conquered the country early in the 16th century and established Mexico as a viceroyalty of New Spain. In 1861, Mexico was invaded by Spain, Great Britain and France. After a period of revolutions, a new constitution was adopted in 1917 providing social reforms. Today, Mexico is a democratic republic of twenty-nine states. There is complete religious freedom with most people Roman Catholic though education is secular, free and compulsory up to the age of fifteen. All church property is vested in the nation but the upkeep of the real estate falls to the clergy.

1. A Michoacan girl in traditional wedding costume of red velvet skirt with green silk border. Green silk capelet with black and white trimming and white fringe. Her yellow felt sombrero is ornamented with roses of varied colors and her slippers are black, worn with white stockings.

2. A Oaxaca woman in her topless turban of thick black woolen yarn, the wearing of which acts as an amulet. The loose ends are left to dangle and occasionally color is added by the threading of red and blue ribbons.

3. The charro or gentleman horseman in a dark blue habit of suède or velvet braided in white. His white felt sombrero is embroidered in gold and silver and his low-cut boots are of soft brown leather. A flowing red silk necktie fastens the collar of his white shirt.

4. A little Tehuan girl wearing the native festival costume which is like that of her elders. In French blue and white, the baby's bodice as well as the woman's blouse are of blue silk. The skirt is white with a band of delicate floral embroidery in shades of blue. Below that, an accordion-pleated frill of fine white lace finished with several rows of "baby ribbon". The huipil grande is also of fine white lace accordion-pleated.

5. A young dandy of Guadalajara wearing an old Spanish costume in black. The jacket is velvet bound with grosgrain ribbon and ornamented with ribbon cockades instead of buttons. Sash and trousers of cloth and a white shirt with colored silk scarf, no doubt scarlet. His felt hat is either beige or gray and the buttoned leather shoes are black.

6. A small Indian boy in white cotton shirt and trousers. A fringed green woolen poncho striped in red and white and a straw sombrero.

7. The traditional Spanish costume of the higher class Mexican woman consisting principally of the mantón, a costly shawl of heavy silk, fringed and richly embroidered in beautiful colors, the high tortoise or ivory comb and handsome earrings. The gown illustrated is dark blue velvet with a golden brown flower at the décolletage. The slippers are black with gold buckles and white stockings.

Mexico

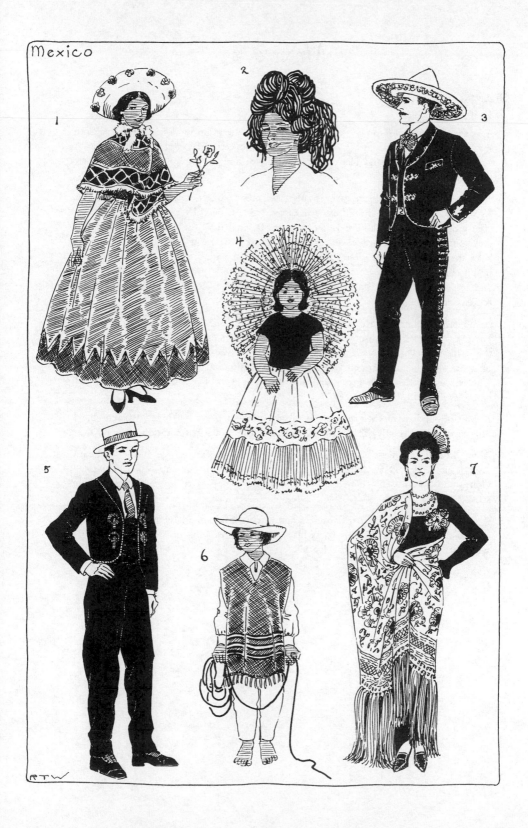

❈ *Mexico* ❈

Plate 70

1. A peon, which may mean a plantation, cattle-ranch or mine worker. The beige cloth suit is tied with a wide, red woolen sash and his neckerchief is red and white silk. A straw sombrero, a red and black serape or blanket and brown leather shoes complete the picture.

2. The festival costume of the women of Tehuantepec worn with the huipil grande. According to legend the headdress was copied from some baby clothes washed ashore after a Spanish shipwreck. The Indian women, fascinated by the dainty pieces, thought they must be feminine headcoverings. They adapted the exquisite little garments into head shawls and thus the design became a traditional part of their holiday dress. The huipil is all-white, of fine cotton and lace and the skirt, a gray blue cotton with band and accordion-pleated frill also of fine white lace. The bodice of dark blue figured silk buttons down the front.

3. A modern version of the costume of the "China Girl" of Old Mexico. She was, supposedly, a princess sold into slavery in Mexico by pirates. In this sparkling creation the darks are red and green motifs appliquéd on a silver-spangled ground. The blouse of white silk, the sash striped green and red on white and a white stripe in the hem. The hair is braided with green, red and white ribbons. The sombrero is yellow felt embroidered with dark red roses.

4. A Mexican Indian mother carrying her baby in the rebozo, a fringed woolen shawl. She wears a dark cloth skirt, a colored cotton apron and a felt sombrero.

5. A tot dressed as a little "country girl" to attend the special service at the Cathedral on Corpus Christi Day. Children also dress as cowboys, priests and nuns. White cap, blouse and apron with colored embroidery. Her ruffled skirt is of blue and white striped cotton.

6. A vaquero or cowboy in black trousers and a fringed blue and white woolen poncho. His sombrero is beige felt, his boots black and he carries the quirt, a favorite riding whip in many Spanish-American locales.

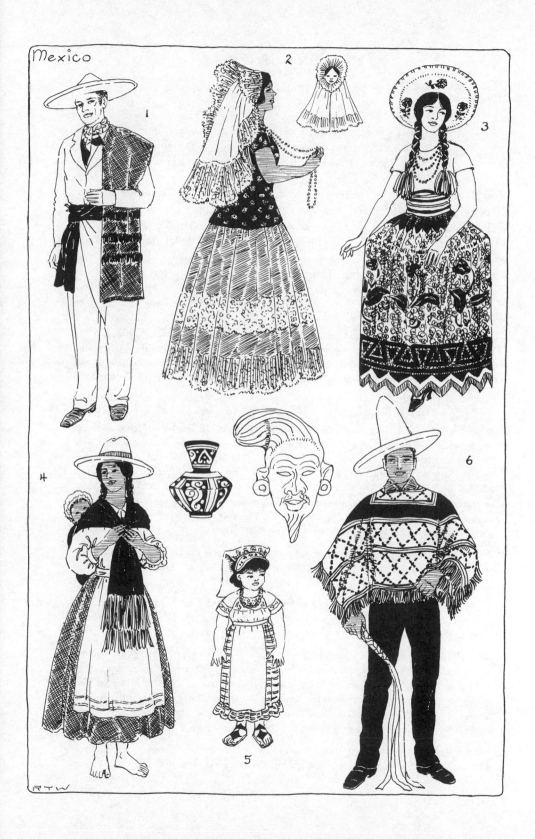

Mexico

1

2

3

4

5

6

RTW

❧ *Mongolia* ❧

Plate 71

Mongolia comprises the Mongolian People's Republic, formerly Outer Mongolia, Inner Mongolia, Tanna and Tuva. Outer Mongolia, one of the oldest countries in the world, was once subject to China. Its people have been nomads lacking historical clarity until the 13th century when the empire began its vast expansion under Genghis Khan. Eventually, the empire reached from China to the Danube in Eastern Europe. In 1924 under Soviet control, the People's Revolutionary was set up. In 1945 a plebiscite declared its independence as the Mongolian People's Republic which was recognized by China in the same year. In Ulan Bator, the commercial and sacred town or capital, are primary and secondary schools and a university. The leading religion is Buddhist Lamaism. Their language is a form or group of kindred languages of the desert or steppe lands of Central Asia.

1. A Buryat-Mongol in tribal dress and a beige felt western hat. His robe or del is a padded silk Chinese brocade in deep rose with a colorful band of embroidery. Underneath, full trousers tucked into his boots of black leather with white-edged soles and peaked toes. The sash is a combination of green and pink and the cuffs are green. The Mongol likes brilliant colors such as shocking pink, royal purple, electric blue and shimmering yellow.

2. This garish costume of everyday dress of the Mongolian woman is from a photograph taken in 1933. The fantastic headdress consists of a gold and silver filigree skullcap worn under the hat. Attached to the cap are two thin horn pieces wound with hair from which hang braids of hair held by jeweled ornaments. The little hat is of fur and tapestry with a metal ornament, the whole arrangement held securely by a strap passing back of the ears and under the chin. The magenta robe is of cloth or velvet and trimmed with fancy braids, one violet, another dark green and an edging of rickrack. Solidly stuffed wings top the sleeves. The soft, red leather peaked-toe boots are embroidered and appliquéd in many colors.

3. An elegant-looking young matron of Chahar in dark blue cotton or cloth and silver jewelry. Her slippers are of dark blue satin worn with white stockings.

4. A woman of Chahar in a costume of "old blue" silk and velvet with an appliquéd white stripe on the bodice. Her cap is of lattice-worked red coral beads with a pendant necklace of red coral beads and gold medallions set with green cabochons. Blue satin slippers with white stockings.

5. Typical Mongolian dress, the padded del in deep rose silk with cuffs of gold-colored velvet and a border of dark blue silk. His fur toque is black, faced with tapestry in shades of yellow. The tiny crown has a jeweled ornament and dark red silk streamers float in back. The hat is secured to the head in the same manner as that of the woman above. Full trousers are tucked into black leather Chinese boots which are roomy enough to take several pairs of stockings in the winter.

6. Buryat-Mongol woman in the traditional padded costume of handsome Chinese silk with woven dragon motifs. A starched white bonnet and her hair in rolled-up braids.

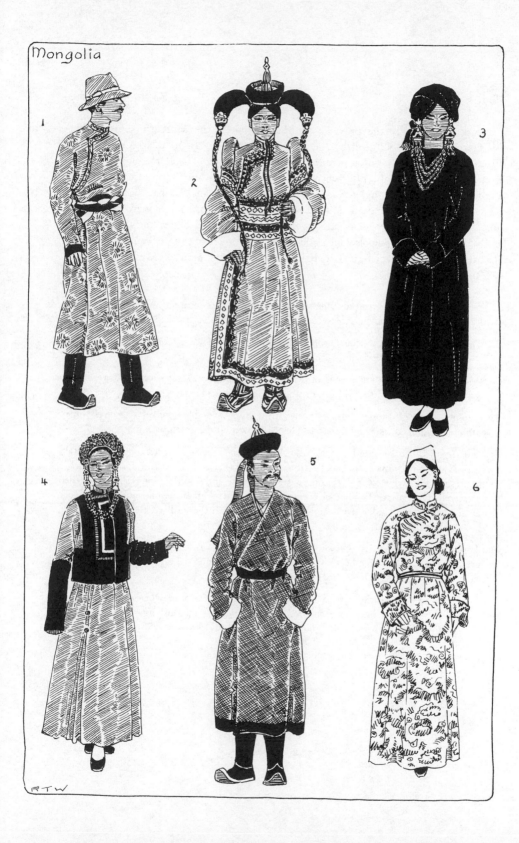

Mongolia

RTW

✶ *Morocco* ✶

Plate 72   see BARBARY STATES

Morocco, originally the province of Mauritania on the southern shore of the Mediterranean, was occupied by the Moslems from the 7th to the 11th centuries. From that time, she has been invaded and held in turn by the Portuguese, Spanish, French and British until 1912 when the greater part became a protectorate of the French. The seaport Tangier was internationalized first in 1925 and again in 1945. In 1962, under a referendum, Morocco became a constitutional monarchy and has accepted aid on a basis of non-interference from the United States, the U.S.S.R. and from France. Trade schools and agricultural training camps are being developed for the population which is largely illiterate. The religion is Moslem and the official language Arabic.

1. A feminine Moslem street costume of caftan, tobe or underdress and djellaba, all in sky blue. The mandeel or face veil of sheer white lawn is finished with embroidery.

2. The crocheted cord cap which is popular among young men worn by itself, is also worn under the headcloth and turban.

3. A favorite haircut of small boys of Fez. The topknot, they say, furnishes a handle by which the wearer, if a Faithful, can be drawn up into Heaven.

4. A combination of Moslem and Western dress in a slate blue tweed and dark blue cotton shirt topped by a red tarboosh. Heavy, brown cordovan shoes.

5. Modern Jewry is permitted to wear the Arab dress. This man is wrapped in several cloaks. The innermost garment of striped cotton is the kumya, a shirt fastened down the front. The wine-colored cotton coat with hood and long flowing sleeves is the farrajiyah. Over that, the short-sleeved gandoura and over all, a burnous of wool or camel's-hair cloth. Under the hood, he wears the gutra, the ends of which hang over the left shoulder for use as needed.

6. Many Moslem women have become emancipated, some discarding the veil, some still covering the chin while others cling to the cover-up custom. This woman of 1960 in her white haik displays her tattoos on forehead and chin.

7. A Moslem boy of wealthy parents in a wine-colored silk burnous worn over the white cotton tobe with pale blue yoke and red embroidery. His tarboosh is of plum-colored felt and the babouches are tooled and colorfully embroidered moroccan leather.

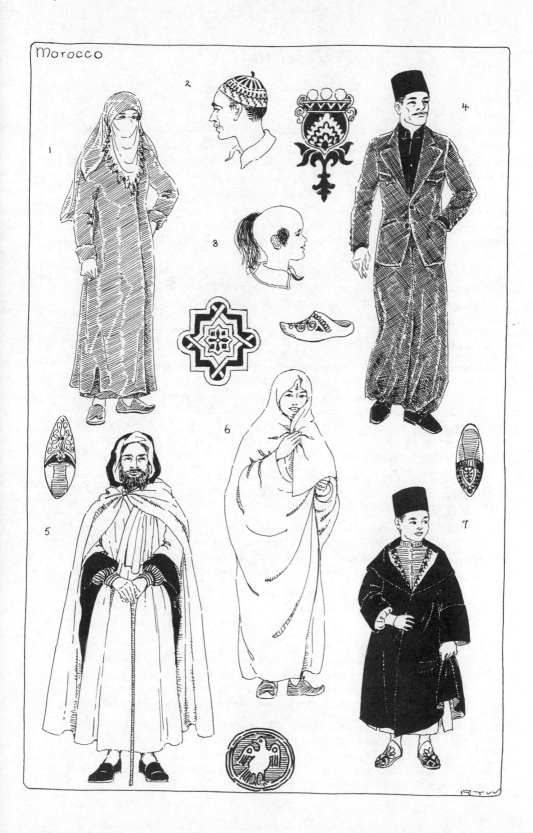

Morocco

❧ *Netherlands* ❧

Plate 73

With the dissolution of Charlemagne's Empire in 814, the Netherlands comprising Holland, Belgium and Flanders split into duchies which were united in the 14th century under the dukes of Burgundy. A revolt against the Spanish branch of the Hapsburgs culminated in 1579 in the seven northern Protestant provinces forming the Union of Utrecht. This led to a declaration of independence in 1581 which was finally recognized in the 17th century. From then on, the Dutch became the commercial nation of Europe. But many upheavals were to erupt, the United Republic ending in 1795, the Belgians in 1850 forming a separate kingdom.

1. A matron of Volendam in the characteristic sheer bonnet of lawn and lace with two outstanding points. The square-cut bodice of the dark blue or brown cloth dress is filled in with an embroidered handkerchief over a vestee of thin flowered woolen cloth. For dress-up occasions many petticoats are worn, six to fourteen of them, and over the outer skirt a very short frilled apron is tied on with a ribbon. The necklace is either coral or amber beads.

2. A starched and wired lace bonnet over a small lawn cap with golden knobs at the temples. Below, a pleated lawn bonnet held in place by "golden horns" indicates the wearer's status, that her husband, brothers and sons of Scheveningen, all are fishermen. In Zeeland women often wear three caps one over the other. The shape of the knobs tell the wearer's religion, round for a Protestant and square for a Roman Catholic. Spiral, corkscrew, gold wire pins with jeweled pendants are worn by the women of various locales. Earrings, too, are a favorite adornment with regional dress.

3. A woman of Zeeland in a broad bonnet of fine lace, starched and wired. Draped over the bodice of her blue or brown dress and tucked into the belt is a vestee of flowered cashmere topped by a coral bead necklace.

4. Both boys and girls wear full skirts and a straight, snug bodice until seven years of age, a boy then changing to the dress of his elders. This young man wears a double-breasted padded jacket colored deep pink with the lower half of the sleeves in a tangerine shade. A dark blue peaked cap, blue socks and sabots, like his father's dress.

5. One of a group off to church on Sunday morning in Middelburg on the island of Walcheren, all wearing the identical costume. Of woolen cloth, probably black, jacket, double-breasted vest and ribbon-bound felt hat. The trousers are secured by a wide leather belt with two large silver rondel buckles.

6. A little maid of Marken whose gown must have been copied from a medieval painting. The skirt is Venetian red velvet edged with blue ribbon. The apron of black velvet has an upper section of Roman striped ribbon. The bodice of white linen is embroidered in muted red and green. An embroidered white linen cap, black stockings and sabots.

7. "Dutchman's breeches", which here are blue, were built for freedom of action on shipboard. The lined cotton jacket is like the boy's above, even to color, a deep pink with forearms of tangerine orange. His knitted dark blue hose are soled with leather, so he can discard the heavy wooden sabots aboard ship. A Paisley printed neck scarf and a handsome black bearskin cap.

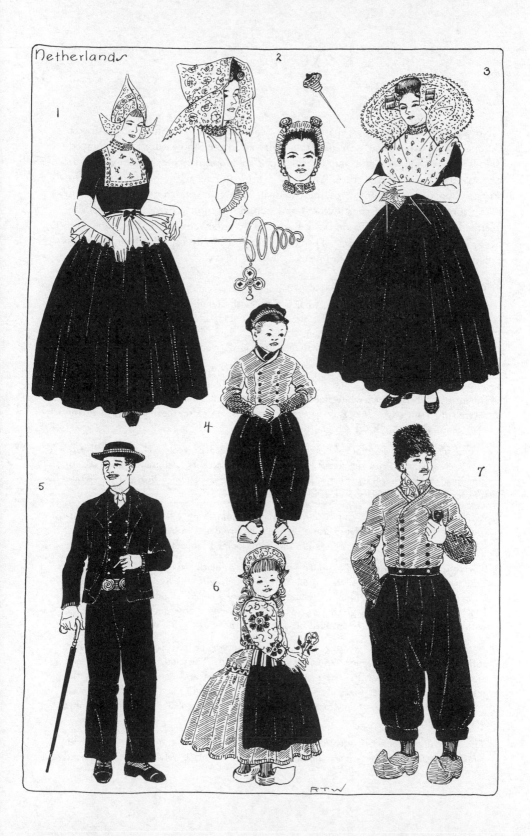

Netherlands

❧ *Norway* ❧

Plate 74

Norway occupies the west part of the Scandinavian Peninsula in northwest Europe. Norse expeditions went out from Norway in the 9th century and colonized islands off Scotland, Iceland and Greenland. The Norsemen became converted to Christianity in the 10th century. There have been unions with the various northern neighbors, the last one with the Swedish Monarchy which was dissolved in 1905. Norway is today a constitutional and hereditary monarchy. All religions are tolerated but that of the Evangelical Lutheran is endowed by the state and the clergy is nominated by the king. The school system, highly organized, makes education compulsory from seven to fourteen.

1. This traditional dress is worn in Setesdal on Sundays and festival occasions. It is fashioned like a pinafore in black woolen cloth with shoulder straps and hemstitched in colorful wool embroidery and worn over the long-sleeved lingerie blouse. The unusual hat looking like an enormous double pincushion is made of silk and ribbon, probably over a wire frame. The handbag is also of woolen cloth with embroidery, and shoes and stockings are black.

2. and 3. Two views of the skaut, the headgear of the Hardanger matron. It is a large square of stiffly starched white linen which is folded, fastened in back and worn in several different ways. The skaut is reminiscent of some of the headgear worn in the 16th century when folk dress began to take hold.

4. The man's festival costume of Setesdal in a heavy black woolen cloth overall embroidered predominantly in scarlet with dark green accents. All motifs are conventionalized in design with further accents of silver. The shirt which boasts a soft white lace-edged collar is of black and white print cotton.

5. A bride of Hardanger wearing a tiara signifying "something old and something borrowed for luck." The corselet of scarlet velvet is embroidered in beads, silver and white. The belt is encrusted with silver as are the hand-loomed lappets of red wool.

6. The traditional dress of a Hardanger bridegroom. A black velvet habit and a scarlet cloth waistcoat, both with silver buttons. Instead of a scarf, this groom wears a silver brooch to fasten the collar of his white linen shirt. The edges of his waistcoat and jacket are handstitched in green yarn. The knitted woolen hose and garters are black with white, worn with silver-buckled black leather shoes.

7. A woman of Telemark wearing traditional costume. The circular cut of the skirt stiffened with circular bands simulates a divided skirt. The cloth trimming is green and scarlet with green cuffs, one green band on the skirt and one on the bodice, the rest being scarlet. Other notes are the lingerie blouse showing at the wrists, the neck and below the very short bolero, a fringed red knitted woolen sash and handsome black leather boots.

8. The Hardanger bonnet, a square headpiece worn by children and young girls. Fashioned of scarlet velvet or woolen cloth, it is edged with black velvet and embroidered with motifs of fine beadwork.

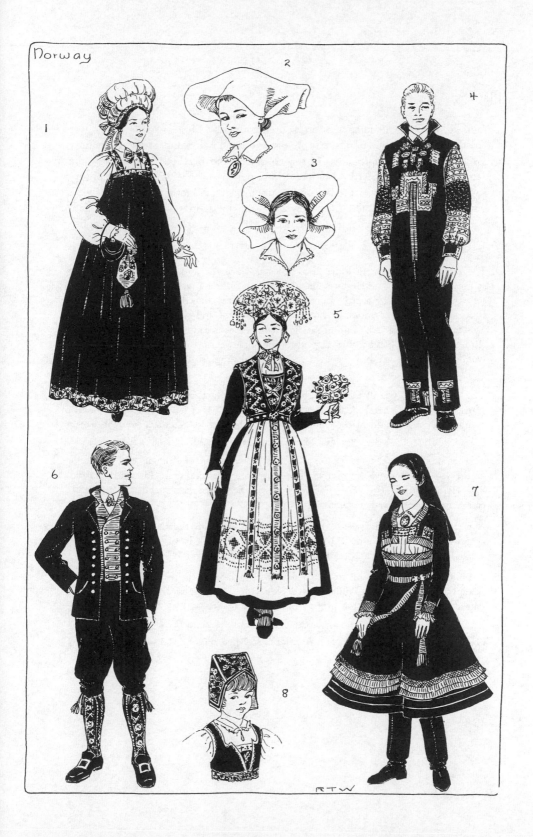

Norway

1

2

3

4

5

6

7

8

RTW

❧ *Pakistan* ❧

Plate 75

Pakistan, a republic composed of a predominantly Moslem population, was founded in 1947, of regions formerly in the Indian Empire under the sovereignty of Great Britain. It occupies areas in the northwest and northeast corners of India which are separated by nearly 1,000 miles. Pakistan shares the 5,000 year-old history of India and is a member of the British Commonwealth. Minorities include Hindus, Christians, Parsees and Buddhists. They have six universities with free and compulsory elementary education the aim. Many languages are spoken but English is official.

1. The sarī has been worn in India, it is believed, since Alexander the Great came and conquered the land. The Hindu woman wears the flattering, artistically bordered scarf, some six yards long by a little more than a yard wide, draped over her left shoulder. It is woven of silk or cotton or both fibers with gold and silver threads. When the Moslem woman wears the Hindu sarī it is composed of cotton with some silk or silk with some cotton because the Koran forbids the wearing of pure silk. The Parsi woman drapes the sarī over the right shoulder to distinguish herself from a Moslem or a Hindu.

2. The wonderful turban of the twenty-four crack cavalrymen of the personal bodyguard of the Governor General. A fine black cloth draped bonnet has a band and cone of orange silk striped with black, white and gold. The stiff black taffeta wing is woven with a narrow dull gold band, the gold threads forming tiny tassels on the edge.

3. The karakul tarboosh worn by this man has been named the "Jinnah cap" in honor of the late Mohammed Ali Jinnah, Pakistan's founder and first Governor General. The cloth jacket is cut long enough to cover the white cotton shirt. Loose white cotton trousers and leather shoes.

4. A merchant who has traveled over the mountains with his camels loaded with merchandise. His worn costume of light brown homespun cloth is sashed with dark green woolen cloth. A fur hat and fur boots, peak-toed and buckled.

5. A Hindu tea picker coming from the field with her basket of tea leaves resting on a headpad. Over a red and white printed blouse or choli, she wears a sarī which is a pale shade of tangerine cotton printed in a deeper shade.

6. An unusual combination of a dark blue choli with a sheer dark green cotton sarī bordered with beige silk. The choli is collared in beige silk and the sandals are brown.

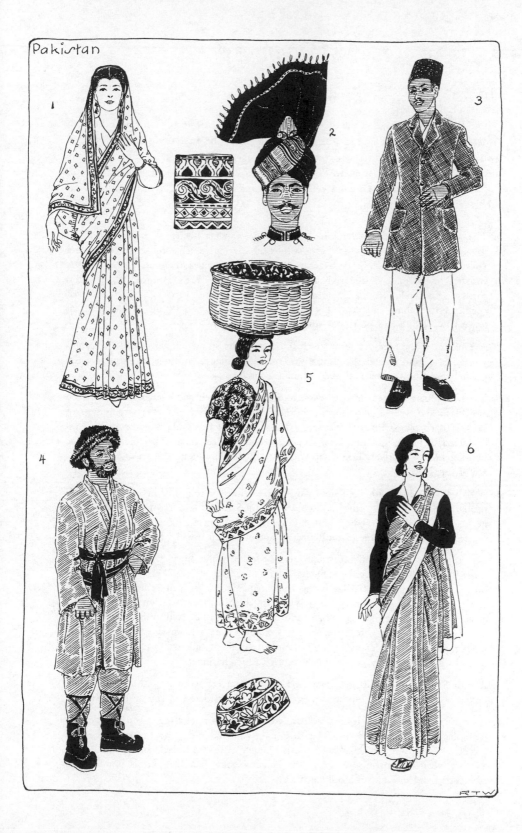

Pakistan

❦ *Panama* ❧

Plate 76

The Republic of Panama on the Isthmus of Panama connects Central and South America. The city of Panama was founded in 1519, the first town to be founded by Europeans on the American continent. It was the chief port for Spanish trade in the 17th and 18th centuries. In 1905, after a revolt from Colombia and recognition from the United States, Panama ceded the Canal Zone to the United States and the canal was completed in 1914.

1. The pollera, the national feminine costume of Panama which is based upon the colonial dress of Spanish ladies, has a waist-deep, flaring capelike collar. Of soft white voile, it is embroidered in deep color such as red or black, here in garnet red. A worsted rosette matches the ribbon sash of dark green. Hand-embroidery, a dozen yards on the bodice and another dozen on the skirt, and yards of fine white lace ruffling finish blouse and skirt. The coiffure is a quivering, sparkling arrangement of flowers, butterflies and pearls on tiny springs.

2. A Guaymi Indian dressed for a festival contest. His straw hat with dark blue and white fabric band is made handsome with macaw plumage, and over a red and white beaded collar, he wears a necklace of hunting souvenirs.

3. San Blas Indian women dress in dark colored cottons such as Chinese red, deep blue and black and wear a gold ring in the nose from babyhood on. This sarong type of skirt is dark blue with violet stripes, and a black blouse with the lower half embroidered in red, yellow and black. Very often the motifs have tribal meanings. The headkerchief is invariably bright red with a printed yellow design. Arm and leg bands are of fine beadwork.

4. A San Blas Indian with gold nose ring and earrings of round, thin gold discs with pendants. Seeds, seashells, silver and gold make up San Blas jewelry, the gold and silver necklaces passed to succeeding generations. Her headkerchief is a red cotton square printed in yellow and orange, and effective accent with a usually dark costume.

5. The masculine Panamanian costume consists of a white linen fringed smock and short breeches hand-embroidered in red, dark blue and yellow. This city man wears brown leather sandals. His hat is the true "panama hat" which is braided and not woven. Braided of palm fibers into a white and black strip, it is sewn and shaped on a wooden block. The fine, smooth, hand-woven "panama" of split and bleached palm-like fibers which grow in Ecuador and Colombia comes from those countries but, having been sold in Panama for more than a century, is called a "panama". In terms of both time and money, it is a much, much costlier headpiece.

6. A little San Blas girl with gold ring in her nose and her wrap-around skirt of polka-dotted black cotton. The blouse is of gray cotton embroidered in red and yellow.

7. A country woman in her festival pollera dress of bright red cotton, a simpler version than that shown in number 1. The skirt has white braiding, the embroidered frills are of white muslin and the décolletage is braided in red and black and finished with a black worsted pompon. She wears the Panama straw hat, her hair is braided and ribbon-tied and she smokes a bulldog pipe.

Panama

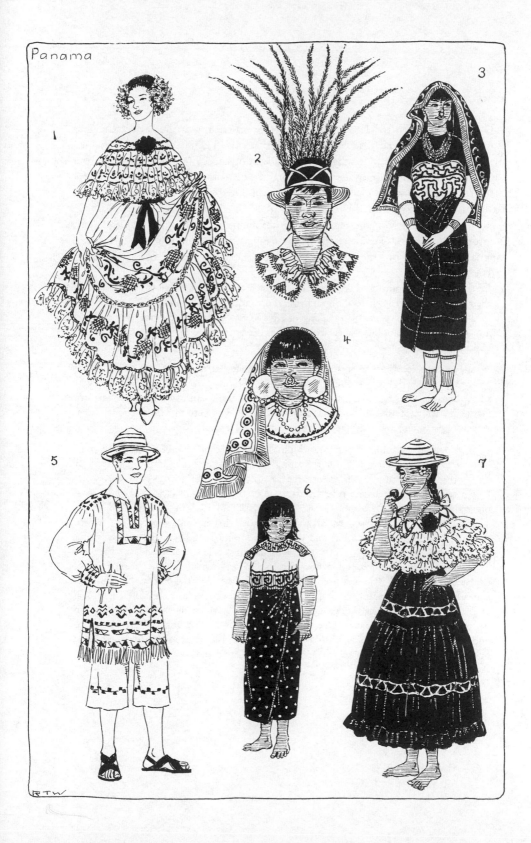

❋ *Peru* ❋

Plate 77

Peru, a republic on the Pacific coast of South America, was the seat of the Inca Empire established about 1250 with Cuzco as its capital. The Spanish arrived in 1522, finally conquering the country by 1533. Rival conquistadors fought each other over the years. In 1542, the viceroyalty of Peru was set up with Lima the seat of government until 1821. Various changes followed until 1923 when it became a republic. Religious liberty is permitted but Roman Catholicism is dominant. Nearly half the population is Indian with the remainder mostly white of Spanish descent and some Negroes, Chinese and Japanese. Elementary education is compulsory. The official language is Spanish but many Indians use their native language.

1. In the Andean countries there are many aristocrats of pure Spanish blood tracing their line of descent back to the grandees who conquered and settled the lands of the Inca Empire. Such a person is this lady in fringed red silk shawl embroidered in black and a black lace mantilla draped over a high, carved tortoise-shell comb worn with a white satin gown.

2. A dashing caballero in leather and velvet. The double bolero is of black and Venetian red velvet with large black silk buttons. A fine white shirt over a black vest with silver buttons. The beautiful cordovan chaparajos or "chaps" are ornamented with black and white braid and laced in front with tasseled thongs. A black felt hat, black velvet breeches and black leather boots complete the ensemble.

3, 4, 5, 6. The love of Incan Indians for pure, brilliant color combined basically with black reflects the influence of their Spanish and Portuguese overlords of yesteryear. Red, green, orange and deep yellow are favorites for embroideries and accessories. Outer skirts and breeches are predominantly black and hats and jackets for both sexes invariably red. Even a wedding dress will be black but sparkling with vibrant color accents. And wool, hand-woven of course, is used in most garments. The serape, number 4, opens down the front and the poncho, number 6, has a hole in the center for the head. On number 4, the square ends hanging below the serape are part of a woolen scarf. The large round hat, which varies in the slant of the brim, is picot-edged and worn by both sexes over a knitted skullcap which ties under the chin. The squarish cap worn in number 6 is peculiar to certain Andean regions. The "coca bag" worn by number 3 carries the leaves of the coca shrub which the natives chew for in-between-snacks and endurance. One side of this bag is knitted with decorative figures and the side shown is sewn with coins. Note also the large silver pins worn by numbers 3 and 5, a fashion which goes back to colonial days.

Peru

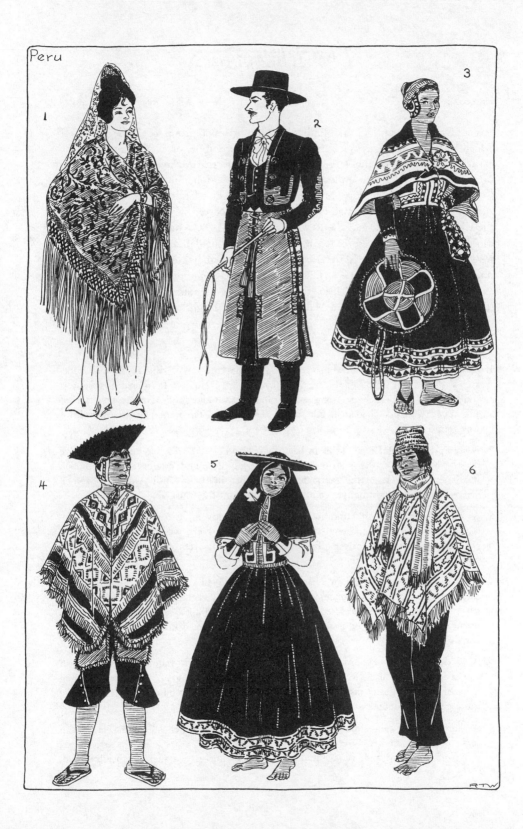

❈ The Philippines ❈

Plate 78   see HAWAII (97)

The Commonwealth of the Philippines comprises a group of 7100 islands of which only 462 have areas of more than a square mile. It is thought that the earliest inhabitants of the largest island group of the Malay Archipelago were Negritoes, followed by the Indonesians and then the Mohammedans who settled in the south in the 15th century. Magellan discovered the islands in 1521 and the first successful settlements were made in 1565. Conflict occurred with Moros in the south, the Chinese, the British and the Revolution of 1896–1899. After the Spanish-American War, the Islands were ceded in 1898 to the United States who paid for the territory. In World War II the Islands were attacked by the Japanese and were under Japanese rule until 1944. The promise in 1934 of independence and set for 1946, was established July 4, 1946. Education is free in public schools. The official language is Filipino based on a Malayan dialect but English and Spanish are commonly used. Roman Catholicism is the religion of most of the people, the remainder being other Christian sects and Moslems.

1. An upper class Philippine woman wearing formal dress with the traditional wide-arched sleeves and fichu. The sleeves and fichu or "pañuelo" are fashioned of rengue, a stiffly starched fabric made from native pineapple. Bodice and skirt or saya are of silk veiled with net plaided in gilt thread. The framed fan is of painted silk with a tiny round mirror.

2. A young girl of the Ifugao Tribe in her tribal costume, each tribe having its distinctive dress. This cotton outfit is striped in black, red, yellow and orange and her pillbox hat is simply a fold of the fabric pinned together in back. Until American women arrived in Luzon, most native women went bare from the waist up.

3. A young woman in the traditional Philippine patadyong costume with the wide-arched sleeves in a plaid rengue or pineapple cloth. Here we have the pañuelo in another style. The clogs or sapatillas may be of anything from cloth, straw or wood to carabao or imported leather.

4. A Moro woman of the sultan's harem, Mindanao, 1940's. Over a chemise of white cotton and breeches of white linen, she wears a silk jacket trimmed with braid and silver buttons. The multicolored striped silk saya is draped about her figure. Her picturesque hat, worn over a silk headkerchief, has a jeweled knob and may be either felt or straw.

5. A workman in a wrap-around cotton skirt striped in red, yellow and black with cotton sash and a black felt tarboosh. Otherwise, the wearing of native dress among the men has practically disappeared with the Western shirt, trousers and jacket being quite generally adopted.

6. A Moro chieftain's daughter with ivory fingernail guards, which means she has harem serfs to wait upon her. Over a white cotton chemise she wears a silk jacket, striped silk pantaloons and a short saya and upon her flowing hair, a tied silk headkerchief.

Philippines

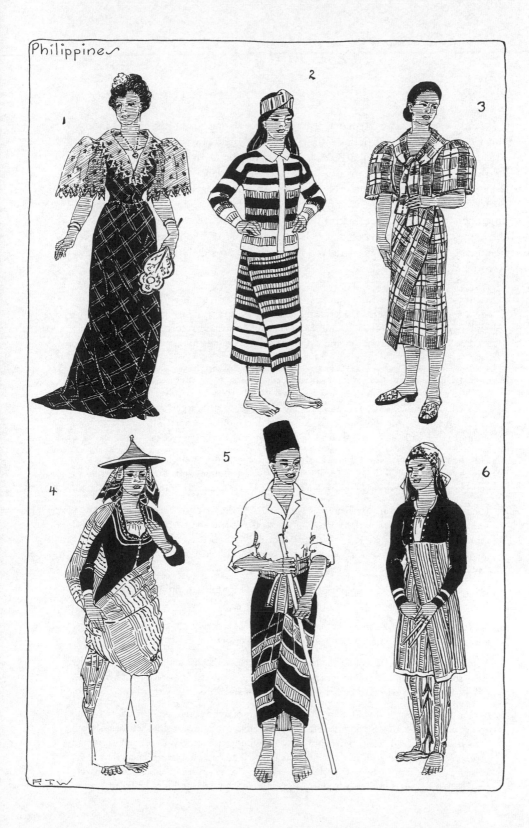

✳ *Poland* ✳

Plate 79   see U.S.A. (98)

Poland, a Communist Republic, has a history dating from the 10th century, and from the 14th to the 17th centuries it was a great power. After 1772, it was successively divided up among Prussia, Russia, Austria, Germany and again Russia. In World War I, it was overrun by the Austrian-German armies. Poland declared its independence in 1918 but in 1939, it was invaded by Nazi Germany and the Soviet Union. In 1947 came complete domination by the Communists despite the opposition of United States and Britain. Education is free and compulsory and there are many institutions of higher learning. Roman Catholicism is the chief religion and complete religious liberty is permitted provided the Church refrains from politics.

1. A man of Kosow in a sheepskin coat worn winter and summer, the wool inside or out according to weather. Underneath, a smock of heavy white linen or homespun with multicolored embroidery and white homespun trousers tucked into white felt bootees. Rawhide carbatines or moccasins laced with thongs and, surprisingly, a straw hat.

2. A bridal costume of Lowicz of brilliant, deep colors, royal blue, green, coral, white and black with narrow multicolored fringe. A black velvet bodice over an embroidered, sheer white cotton blouse. A wonderful headdress of fresh flowers, white with touches of pink, and around her neck, white coral and amber beads. Soft black leather bottines laced with blue ribbons over pink stockings.

3. The men of Zduny wear this dark blue cloth jacket, silver-buttoned, with sleeves or sleeveless over a white linen shirt. The black striped orange cloth breeches are tucked into black leather boots. The black felt pork pie hat is encircled with a narrow ribbon.

4. The women of Żabie are excellent equestriennes and when riding, wear such a costume. The sheepskin sleeveless jacket, here worn with the fur to the inside, accompanies two aprons of homespun cloth striped in shades of red, one in back and one in front. The chemise, which is blouse and underskirt, is of white linen or homespun belted with a colorful girdle. Embroidered felt boots and a silk headscarf.

5. The bridal headdress of a groom of Kraków. A black skullcap dressed with pink and white flowers and peacock feathers for good luck.

6. A little tot of Sokoloka in a sleeveless sheepskin jacket gayly embroidered. His white shirt and breeches are of heavy linen or woolen homespun.

7. Another young man of Sokoloka, also in a sleeveless sheepskin jacket over a white linen smock and breeches. He wears leather leggings tucked into laced leather shoes. A knitted hat of variegated colors with a knitted band threaded with ribbon.

8. A man of Kraków in his Sunday dress. A capote of white homespun with red cloth lining and lapels and black tassel fasteners. Undercoat and breeches of black cloth with red piping and front pieces and pockets, white with red. White linen shirt and silver buttons on the coat and the black felt hat. The breeches are tucked into black leather boots and held by a wide leather belt with a large ornamental plaque. Every man makes his own leather belt and plaque studded with large brass nailheads.

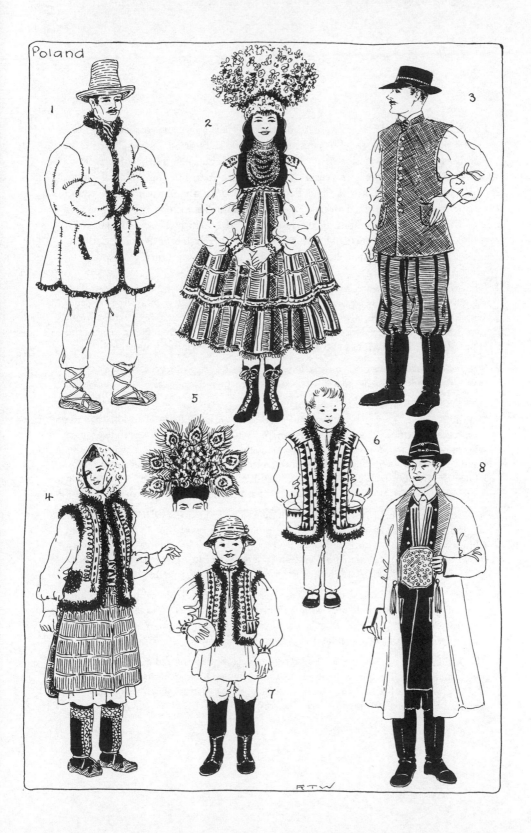

Poland

RTW

✳ *Portugal* ✳

Plate 80

Portugal occupies the western part of the Iberian Peninsula in Europe. The ancient inhabitants were the Lusitanians who were subjugated by the Romans in the 2nd century, by the Visigoths in the 5th century and later by the Moors. They expelled the Moors in the 13th century and became a maritime and colonial power in the 15th and 16th centuries. The Portuguese opened the African coast, found the Cape route and colonized Brazil. Portugal became the European trading center but gradually lost much empire to the Dutch and the British. It was proclaimed a republic in 1910, is now actually a dictatorship. The religion is Roman Catholic, religious freedom is tolerated and primary education is compulsory.

1. The women of Minho are known for charm, beauty and artistry in their dress. This costume is basically wine red and faded dark blue. Bodice and skirt are red bordered with red. A soft, white lawn blouse with a neck frill and the apron, a mixture of blue, red and dull green tied with blue strings. An embroidered fabric pouch and slippers with white stockings and the headkerchief silk in wine red and rose.

2. The men's Madeiran festival costume of white shirt and baggy breeches with a fringed sash also of linen. Yellow goatskin boots and the "pigtail" cap called carapuça. The men prefer black for ceremonial dress.

3. One of a group of women of Esposende and neighboring villages who all wear the same everyday dress. They walk down on the sand to the shore to meet their men who have spent the day fishing. They wear a pink cotton skirt with a white blouse, a red or green knitted woolen shawl and a black woolen shawl tied about the hips. Under the coquettish black felt hat, a colorful silk headkerchief and on the hat in front, a sparkling tiny mirror, presumably to flash a welcoming signal in the sun.

4. A picturesque shepherd in dark blue and brown. The knitted Phrygian bonnet, sleeveless jacket, sash and trousers are blue. The quilted bolero with sleeves is of blue and white checked cotton with blue braiding. Over the trousers are worn chaps of brown sheepskin and on his feet, laced brown leather shoes. Over his right shoulder he carries a folded brown cloth blanket which is lined with the blue and white checked cotton.

5. Madeira's traditional festival women's costume of red cloth striped with black, white, blue and yellow and a red cape worn as illustrated. The edges of cape and skirt are bound with yellow. Over the white blouse, a corselet laced in front. Women, as do the men, wear the black pigtail cap and yellow goatskin boots.

6. The regional dress of a man of Aveiro. A sleeveless jacket of red cloth with white border and large silver buttons with black braid frogs or Brandenburgs. A red, fringed silk sash with the black cloth trousers and laced black leather shoes. His traditional hat has a black velvet brim with black silk crown.

Portugal

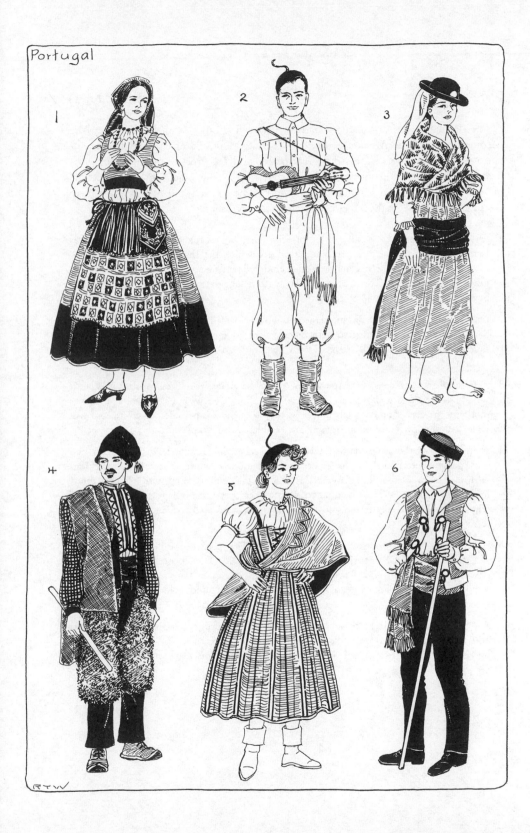

❧ *Pyrenees* ❧

Plate 81   see U.S.A. (102)

The Pyrenees form a natural barrier between France and Spain from the Mediterranean to the Atlantic, setting the Iberian Peninsula apart from the rest of Europe. This barrier is traversed by few passes and has crossings only at the ends near the coast. French engineers, early in our century, built a good road but because of winter snows, it is a seasonal thoroughfare. The French and Spanish in native costume attend the festivals held in each other's villages.

1. A young woman of Castillon who prefers Paris styles for everyday wear to this family-heirloom costume. Bonnet and shawl are white, the shawl embroidered in stylized red roses. A plaid silk apron is blue and red and her woolen skirt is striped in gray and dark blue. The wooden sabots with exaggerated peaked-toes surely must be the most uncomfortable of all footwear.

2. One of a group of 2000 Basque dancers who performed in the Spanish bull ring at San Sebastian. Red cloth bolero with black velvet edge and breeches. White shirt and faja or sash of white silk striped with red and green. Black slippers and white stockings.

3. A Catalonian dancer visits the festival in Amélie-les-Bains. Her dress is black silk with white lace and fine white voile. The apron is embroidered with a large colorful flower motif in one corner and a small flower in the other. The cap is also of white lace and voile and her straw-colored alpargatas are beribboned in deep pink.

4. A farmer in Bethmale in dark blue denim breeches and brown leather leggings tied with gayly colored, tasseled woolen strings. His modern white shirt collar is also tied with tasseled woolen strings. Over his bright red sash embroidered with a wheat motif in yellow, he wears a tan knitted jacket with embroidery done in black, red and yellow. The jaunty knitted cap is red and yellow and the very old wooden sabots date back to medieval days.

5. An elaborate festival dress of a Bethmale woman. The black in the illustration signifies red, a soft red with braid trimming of black and gold. The upper part of the bodice is white printed with pink flowers. An underskirt of muted purple plaided in yellow. White sleeve frills and white bonnet with black crown and gold ribbon band, and wooden sabots.

6. A Catalonian dancer in black velvet festival dress with brilliant red sash and cap. Red and white side stripes and yellow fringe adorn his breeches. He wears a red silk neckerchief and carries a tambourine in his hand. With his black stockings he wears alpargatas with deep pink stitching and gartering.

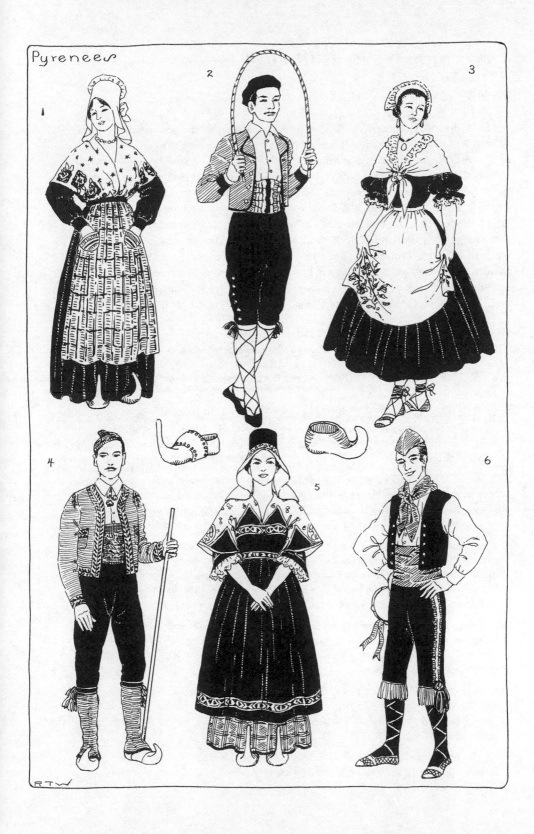

Pyrenees

❧ *Rumania* ❧

Plate 82

The history of Rumania, a Balkan state, precedes the merged peoples of the Dacian Kingdom by centuries. Rome occupied the Dacian Kingdom from 101 A.D. to 274 A.D. In our time the principalities of Wallachia and Moldavia, dominated by Turkey, united in 1859, becoming Rumania in 1861. Rumania regained complete independence from Turkey in 1878 and helped Russia against Turkey in the Russia-Turkish War of 1877–1878. She entered World War I on the side of the Allies. Under the regime of Antonescu in World War II, Rumania was forced to join Germany against the U.S.S.R. and was then overrun by Russia in 1944. She was proclaimed a Peoples' Republic in 1947. Primary education is free and compulsory. The language is founded on Latin with influences of French, Greek, Slav and Turkish. Freedom of religion is assured but the Greek Orthodox Church has been absorbed by the state and the Roman Orders have been abolished.

1. A peasant of Transylvania in his Saturday night "dress-up". A black cloth sleeveless jacket and a black cloth or felt coat beautifully embroidered in toned-down rich colors. Smock and breeches of heavy white linen with a sash of color. A black felt hat with a posy tucked into the ribbon band. Brown rawhide shoes and brown knitted woolen leggings.

2. With her hair in braids, her tall hat denotes maidenhood among the Saxon girls of Transylvania in Rumania. Her costume combines black velvet and white lawn or voile, lace-trimmed. Skirt, corselet, cape and hat are black. A square silk scarf is fastened at her waist.

3. A man of Bukovina in a white sheepskin waistcoat, a style worn also by the women. It is bordered with black lamb and the floral motif is embroidered in many gay colors. Bright blue is the color of the embroidery on his white linen smock and his sash may be blue or black. White linen trousers and laced brown leather shoes.

4. The unmarried girl wears a bright silk bandana, this one orange, whereas the young matron dresses her head in a scarf of silk veiling. The black velvet bolero and the fine black homespun apron are both embroidered in black and gold, the apron edged with black crocheted lace. Blouse and skirt are of sky blue cotton with an embroidered hem. A Roman-striped silk sash, black slippers and white stockings.

5. A young man off to church in his Sunday dress. The white sheepskin coat is embroidered in brown and rust and edged with a picot trimming of rust felt. Black or brown fur collar and lining and a hip pocket on each side toward the back. Hat, trousers and shoes are black.

6. A young woman in white blouse and skirt, the blouse decorated with simple geometrical designs in red and black. The black woven apron is ornamented with black crochet lace and the sash is of silk striped orange and black. Orange, too, is the color of her headkerchief.

At the top of the page is a good example of Rumanian unconventionalized design from a colorful rug border of the mid-19th century.

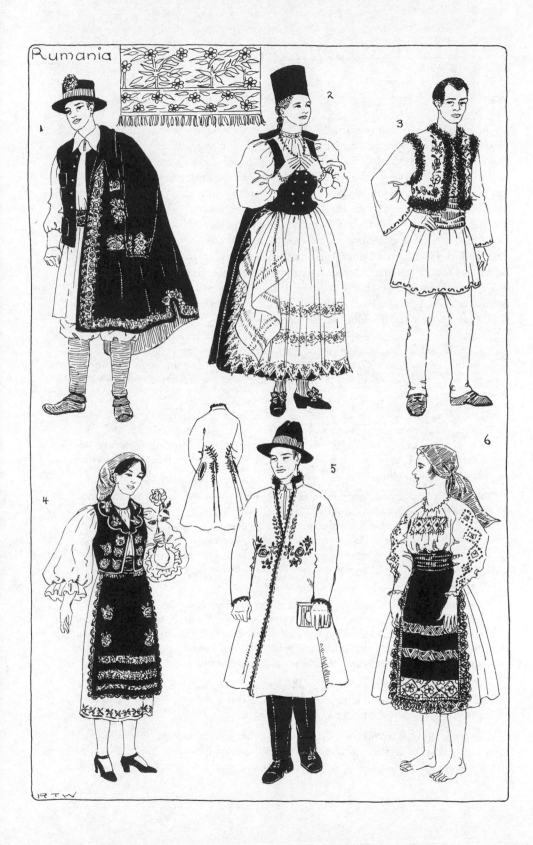

Rumania

✳ *Russia* ✳

Plate 83   see ARMENIA, ESTONIA, U.S.A. (98)

From the 5th to the 8th centuries A.D. Russia was settled by the Eastern Slavs and in the 9th century by Scandinavians who established Novgorod and Kiev. Russia was invaded by the Mongols in the 15th century. From the 14th and 15th centuries as the princes of Moscow acquired power, they began the defeat of the Tatars, overran and annexed rival principalities and advanced against the Ottoman Empire. In 1867 Russia sold Alaska to the United States. She entered World War I with the Allies 1914–1917, overthrew the czarist regime in 1917 and after the Bolshevist Revolution, set up a government of soviets. The first constitution was adopted in 1918 and in 1922, Russia joined the other soviet republics to form the Union of Soviet Socialist Republics. Universal compulsory education was decreed in 1930. More than a hundred languages are taught. In 1918, the separation of Church and State took effect. Christianity is represented by nine branches of the Orthodox Church with Islam, Jewish and Buddhist faiths following.

1. A Kazakh chief in a magnificent coat of snow leopard, a large leopardlike cat which inhabits the high altitudes of Tibet and South Siberia. It is gray or cream color marked with brown rosettes. His cap is of red fox and his black boots are fashioned of soft leather.

2. A "shepherdess" of Kirghiz wears this costume tending the livestock, which may be a herd of yak. Her caftan is of quilted cotton, red with a white floral design. Underneath, a linen smock over pantaloons tucked into boots. The boots are dark blue with white soles and appear to be of dyed sheepskin with the wool to the inside. The tall bonnet or calpac is of white felt with brides of felt and strings of beads. Long strings of beads also hang round her neck.

3. This man of Uzbek is dressed for travel in a striped caftan with a silk square folded diagonally and tied round the waist. Like the Turkish gutra, it is probably used as headkerchief, handkerchief and what not. His pantaloons are tucked into leather boots and his jaunty cap is studded with colored stones. The cap is called a tyubetevka, a Uzbek fashion which is worn all over Central Asia and has been taken up by the Russians. This costume is in strange contrast to his means of transportation, which is often a plane.

4. A Latvian woman in a coat of white homespun or sheepskin with the wool to the inside. Sleeves, fringe, banding and embroidery are red. A blue skirt and a fringed, hand-loomed woolen apron done in red and yellow. Red and white is the color scheme of the bonnet which is a tarboosh draped with silk. The hanging plaques in back are fringed and embroidered with cross-stitching. Late 19th century.

5. A skilled worker of Moscow in his Sunday clothes. The suit is of dark cloth with a double-breasted vest over the white linen smock. Favored colors are dark green, dark blue and brown. A peaked cap and black leather boots.

6. A gypsy of Irkutsk in Siberia. Her blouse is of white linen and the skirt of flower-printed cotton. Over the ensemble, a black silk apron edged with lace and banded with ribbon. She wears earrings, strings of beads, a bright colored headkerchief and black leather slippers.

Russia

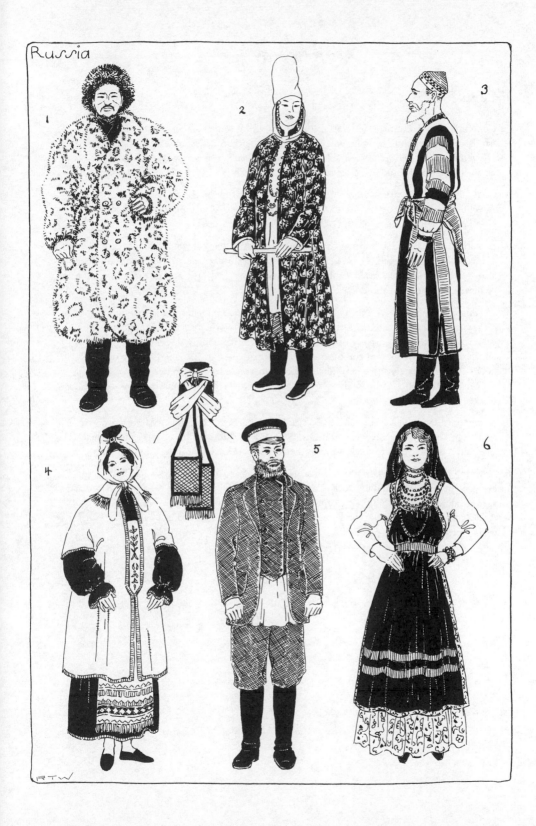

❦ *Russia* ❦

Plate 84

1. Contemporary Ukrainian festival costume. A white linen smock with embroidered bands on sleeves and hem in green and yellow with touches of green and red and a fringed sash of red and green silk. The sleeveless jacket of white linen is edged with black lamb's wool and embroidered in black.

2. Contemporary festival costume worn in the Youth Parade in Lenin Stadium, Moscow. A yellow cotton dress with brown ribbon trimming. A Venetian red velvet sleeveless jacket sewn with white paillettes and white ribbon. Red leather boots.

3. A native of Kabardino in the Caucasian Mountains late in the 19th century. His dolman-sleeved cloak is gray blue cloth with gold braid and the trousers are dark blue also finished with gold braid. A fur calpac, probably fox, and all the trappings of a well-armed traveler in those days.

4. An Armenian woman of Van in the late 19th century. Her chalwar or pantaloons are of rose-colored satin and so is the yelek, a garment worn over the pantaloons. This yelek buttons to the waist, is open at the sides from the hips down and has sleeves which show below those of the outer robe. Another yelek of brocaded cashmere visible down the front, is sleeveless and also open down the sides. The outer robe is of light brown cloth and her tarboosh is wrapped round with a folded square of figured silk. Peaked-toed rose satin slippers.

5. A shepherd tending Karakul sheep on a collective farm in Turkmen. Cloth pantaloons and dolman-sleeved robe with braid trim, a linen shirt, leather boots and a black sheepskin bonnet, all of which, despite the fur cap, must be summer apparel.

6. A young woman of Uzbek attired in a gayly patterned and brilliantly colored cotton or woolen robe. Her "bobby socks" and canvas shoes signify mild weather. Women, as well as men, wear the Uzbek cap, the tyubetevka which is popular all over Central Asia and has been taken by the Russians. Like the man in Plate 83, she wears this outfit even when traveling by plane.

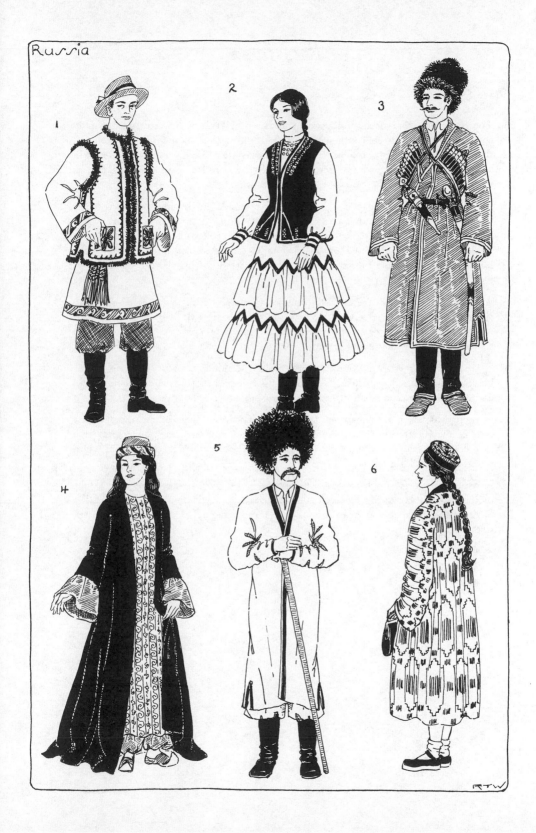

Russia

1

2

3

4

5

6

RTW

❊ *Russia* ❊

Plate 85

1. The rich dress of a woman of Kazan in the late 19th century. The caftan is of gold-colored brocade with gold satin border and girdle over a sheer white blouse. The sleeves are lined with rose-colored satin. The underskirt is French blue with gold satin hem and the overskirt of moss green velvet. Her headdress is a square of brocade in variegated colors and she wears soft leather papushes.

2. The contemporary traditional costume worn by several Asiatic republics of the U.S.S.R. This was worn in a Youth Parade in Lenin Stadium, Moscow. Bright dark green cloth tunic trimmed with red and yellow braid. Leather belt with a large silver buckle. White shirt with embroidered and tasseled collar tabs. Red cloth breeches and black leather boots with white cuffs striped in red and black and fringed with red tassels. A red fox cap.

3. A dancer of Caucasia of the late 19th century. Her jacket is of wine-colored silk with silver banding worn over a white lawn or silk underbodice which is sewn with silver coins. An olive green silk skirt. The draped turban is fashioned of Bayadere striped silk with a filmy white veiling in back.

4. A farmer in Daghestan in Caucasia in his white sheepskin coat set off smartly by his black woolen shirt or rubashka. He is wearing full pleated pantaloons, woolen socks and rawhide shoes and a handsome black sheepskin bonnet.

5. A young woman in Ukrainian festival costume. The white linen blouse and skirt are lavishly embroidered in floral colors. Apron in black woolen homespun embroidered in red, green, yellow and white with a sash of black and white checked cotton edged with black. Red leather boots.

6. A wealthy native of Bukhara who fled the city in the 1920's when it became a state of the U.S.S.R. His richly brocaded robe or caftan is in wine and gold color with a handsome buckled leather belt. A skullcap of moroccan red leather with a narrow silk braid.

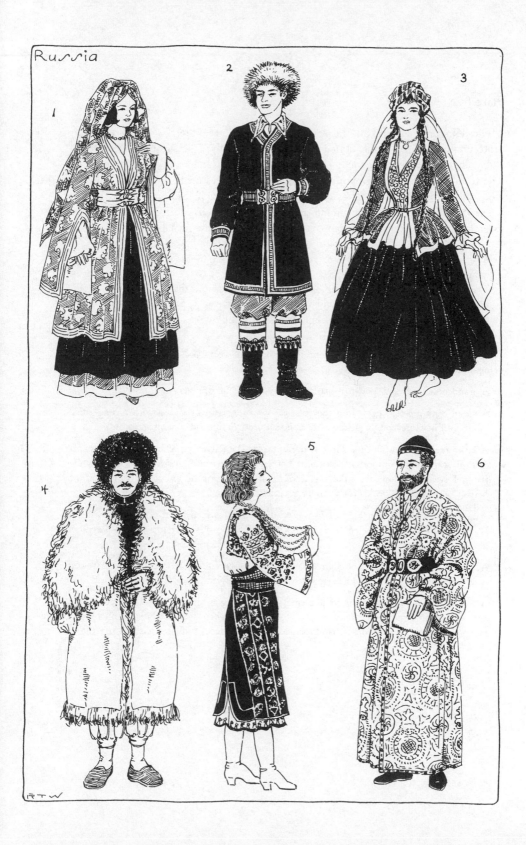

Russia

1

2

3

4

5

6

RTW

❧ *Sikkim* ❧

Plate 86

The Kingdom of Sikkim, formerly a British protectorate, is now an Indian protectorate. Situated in the Himalayas it is bordered by Tibet, Bhutan, Nepal and India and is the shortest route between India's plains and the Tibetan plateau. The true Sikkimese or original inhabitants were cream-skinned Lepchas and Bhotias who came from Tibet centuries ago. They were settled in Sikkim by the British when the British ruled India. Buddhism is their religion. As to language, there are several Himalayan dialects spoken but English is now the official language.

1. A prince in his wedding dress of gold cloth exquisitely brocaded in black, red and white. The undergarment of fine white linen or cotton shows at the neck and sleeves. The long sleeves are evidence of his high status and show that he need not work. His footwear is black with red and white motifs. The cap is black velvet with a silk crown of yellow and Chinese blue topped with a coral button.

2. A beautiful hat of gold-colored velvet embroidered in soft colors and brimmed with mink or sable. Her black hair is braided and she wears a necklace of coral, black agate and pearl beads.

3. A handsomely draped sari in a brocade of violet silk and silver.

4. A small Sikkimese princess in a robe of peacock blue satin brocaded with a blue-green motif and a white cotton jacket with a varicolored design on a white ground.

5. A custom unique to Sikkim, Tibet and Bhutan is the exchange of ceremonial or benediction scarfs upon important occasions between friends and guests. The pure white fringed scarf of cotton or silk is placed upon the palms of an older or important person or round the neck of a younger recipient.

6. A brocaded white wedding gown in the wrap-around, draped baku of Lepcha women. It is secured with a jeweled belt hung with gold and silver chains and a Lepchan dagger.

7. A young prince in a baku of orange satin brocade with sash of deeper crêpe. His cap is of yellow satin brocaded in beige with orange bands and a coral button on top.

8. A village woman proceeding to a cremation carrying a prayer wheel, prayer beads and a black umbrella. Her baku is of gray-blue cloth worn over a white cotton blouse. Her colorful, woolen apron is hand-loomed in three pieces which are sewn together.

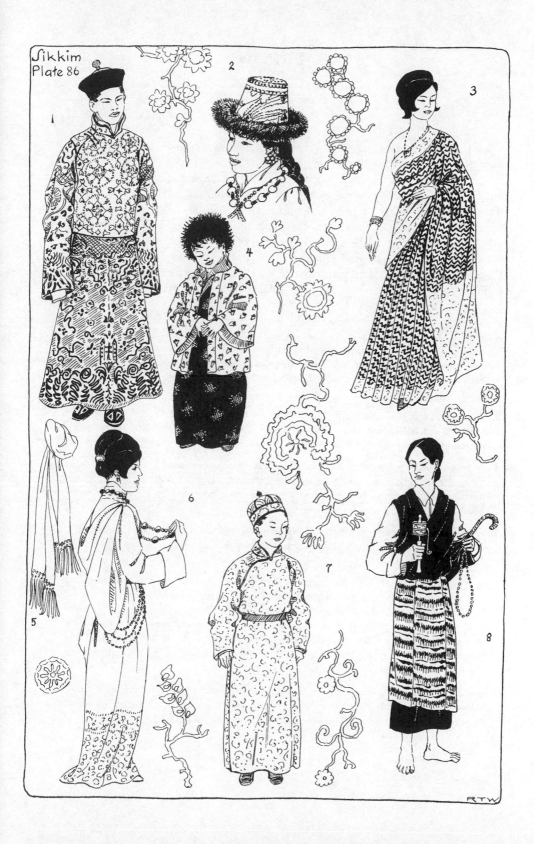

❧ *Spain* ❧

Plate 87

see BALEARIC ISLANDS, CANARY ISLANDS,
GYPSIES, PYRENEES

Spain is a nominal monarchy, although without a monarch, and except for Portugal, occupies the entire Iberian Peninsula. It was settled by the Iberians, Basques and Celts and conquered by Rome in 200 B.C. Spain adopted Christianity but by 711 A.D. was conquered by the Islamic invasion from Africa. The Moors were driven out during the reign of Ferdinand and Isabella in the same year that Columbus discovered America for Spain. With the conquest of Mexico, Peru and other colonial expeditions, she acquired a great empire. After political upheavals and revolution in the 1930s, General Franco was installed as Chief of State. In language, Castilian is spoken by more than two-thirds of the people, Basque in the north, Galician in the northwest and along the Mediterranean, Catalan.

1. A woman of Segovia in the twentieth century wearing a peasant costume of old Seville. The bolero is a rich dark blue silk with red bowknots at the shoulders. Girdle and skirt are of red cloth, an ivory buckle, and black velvet ribbon and stitchery on the skirt. Apron and bonnet are black, the bonnet ornamented with gold embroidery, dark blue ribbon and a red tuft. The fine white lace mantilla is tucked into the décolletage and a bead necklace rests on the bosom.

2. A woman of Seville wearing the Andalusian comb of tortoise shell with yellow satin bowknot and red carnations, a white hibiscus blossom and a "Manila shawl" of white silk embroidered in brilliant colors.

3. A peasant of Mogarras in fiesta dress. The felt cap, capa or cloak, jacket, shirt, vest, wide sash or faja, pantaloons and leggings, all in dark blue cloth except his white linen collar. The bolero is gathered to a narrow yoke front and back in smock style. The vest is buttoned with large silver nuggets.

4. A man of Turégano in fiesta dress. Felt sombrero, cloak, jacket, sash and breeches, all of black cloth. The shirt and stockings are white with alpargatas or hempen sandals in black and white.

5. A woman of Montehermoso in western Spain where in the late 1930's regional costume was still worn as everyday dress and where the elaborate piece of work passes from mother to daughter. The dress is of black cloth as are the many petticoats. The skirt is shaped by fine shirring or tucks over an exaggerated dome-shaped form, the whole made colorful by brilliant machine-made ribbons. The bonnet is of gauze and fine lace over a silk cap and the high boots are gayly embroidered or appliquéd with pieces of dyed leather.

6. A young woman of Murcia in her fiesta dance costume of Chinese red with heavy white cotton embroidery. The overskirt is edged with white and her fringed silk shawl is pure white. Red silk stockings with white slippers add a flashing note.

Spain

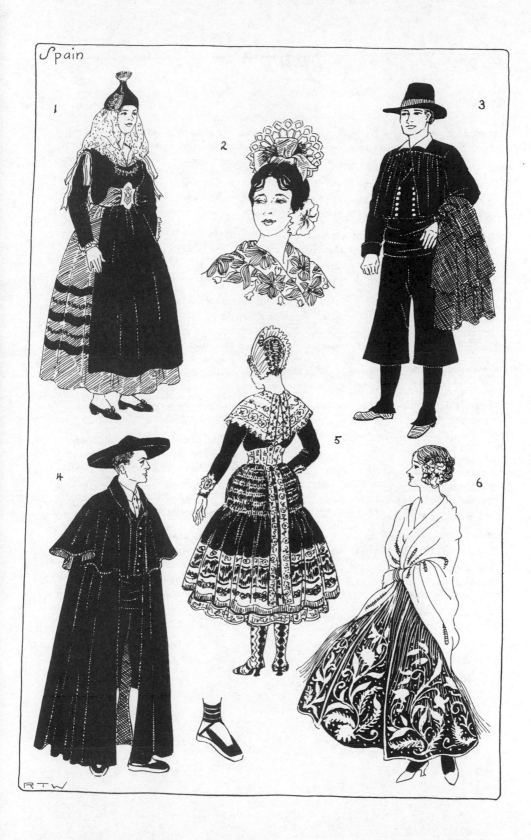

Spain

Plate 88

1. A woman of Turégano in a formal and handsome scarlet velvet fiesta gown ornamented with gold passementerie. Gold stitchery outlines the décolletage and the piccadills of the bodice. The scarlet velvet cap is adorned to match.

2. A man of Salamanca in one of the many distinctive peasant styles of that locale. This bolero is of velvet in brown, dark blue or black and embroidered in a floral design of delightful colors. He wears the wide sash and a felt hat with ribbon band.

3. A "fastidious" gypsy, one of a group of cave-dwellers in Purullena, Andalusia. His velvet hat, cloth sash, breeches and leggings are black. The jacket is of red velvet with braided edge and tasseled braid ornaments. The white frilled shirt is set off by a black silk neckband. Carried on one leg is what appears to be a hunting knife.

4. A torero in his spectacular costume of gold and silver brocade and embroidery combined with black velvet and overlaid with tasseled squares. The capa of heavy cherry-colored satin is lined with yellow silk. The silk stockings are pink and the firm leather slippers are black. The cap which is unique to bull-fighting is shaped like a skullcap with stubby horns that are weighted, making the cap a heavy headpiece. The top is cloth decorated with a stylized motif of a bull's eye in black braid and the body is covered with tufted black cloth which gives the effect of black Persian lamb. At center back at the edge of the cap he wears a black ribbon cockade with a tiny turned-up queue.

5. A young woman of Lagartera of the Province of Toledo in fiesta ceremonial dress. Of black silk with a yoke of black silk crocheted lace. The laced bodice is orange with embroidered pink trim which is also used on the skirt to simulate an apron. The balloon-shaped sleeves are lined with a stiffener and finely shirred. The dome-shaped section is tucked over a foundation. Her stockings are flesh-colored with flower embroidery and her high shoes are elaborately embroidered or appliquéd.

6. A Spanish peasant of the south of Spain whose traditional and elaborate costume reveals centuries of Moorish influence. All the many colors are in muted tones on black, resulting in an artistic piece of work. Gold fringe borders the fichu and the wine-colored satin flounce of the apron. The delicately embroidered, sheer white mantilla and the fine handkerchief add to the formality of the creation. White stockings and embroidered slippers.

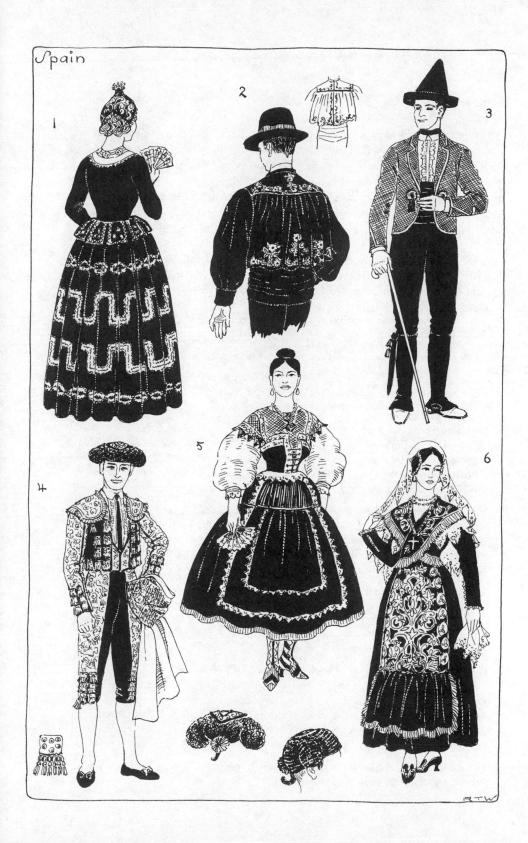

Spain

❊ Sweden ❊

Plate 89

The history of Sweden, a Germanic people, begins with Viking raids in the 9th century. They became united and converted to Christianity in the 11th century. The Swedes conquered the Finns in the 12th century and in the 14th century, united with Denmark and Norway. Breaking with the House of Vasa, they began a vast territorial expansion and by the 17th century, had become the leading Baltic power. Much of her territory was lost in the following centuries. She became a constitutional monarchy in 1809, Norway entering into union with her 1814–1908.

1. A young woman of Dalecarlia. Her skirt and corselet are of black wool cloth, the corselet laced with red ribbons into silver hooks. The apron is dark blue. Over the white linen blouse, she wears a fringed shawl heavily embroidered on a red ground. The same embroidery appears on the hem of the skirt and ornaments the black cloth pouch and bonnet. Red stockings and black slippers.

2. A young woman of Rättvik wearing a tall pointed bonnet of black velvet with a headband of twisted black and white ribbon and a red bowknot at the nape.

3. A young woman of the Dal Region in a red bonnet with a roll framing the face and a ruffle in back. A twisted black and white ribbon headband ends in red ribbon ties. A front view is shown above.

4. A man of Dalecarlia wearing chamois-colored suède breeches and a red suède waistcoat with red buttons. A green ribbon fastens the soft turn-over collar of his embroidered white linen shirt. His green felt hat is banded in red. Yellow and green knitted woolen garters secure the knitted white wool hose accompanied by brown leather shoes with square tongues.

5. A woman of Södermanland Province wearing a leather-belted green cloth apron over her red cloth dress. Simple embroidery stitches adorn the apron. There is an embroidered yellow bodice over the white linen blouse. Her cap resembles that of Norway, being a stiffly starched square of linen fastened and puffed to her fancy. Red stockings and black leather boots.

6. An older man of Delebo in a habit, the design of which goes back centuries. His cassock and breeches are of dark blue cloth, the coat piped in red and worn with a red suède waistcoat piped in green, the two garments well supplied with brass buttons. A knitted red "liberty cap," knitted blue hose and knitted red wool garters with blue motifs and black leather shoes.

7. The pointed bonnet worn here is of starched white muslin with a narrow face frill. The young woman wears a green cloth bolero piped with yellow over a white muslin blouse. Skirt and apron are made in one, simulating the traditional apron of homespun. The back section is black velvet with the front of striped silk in Chinese red, black and gold, the hem matching this latter. The pouch on a chatelaine belt is of embroidered homespun in white, pale rose and green, stockings red and slippers black.

8. The same bonnet as that shown on number 1, of red velvet or cloth with wool embroidery in black, green and yellow.

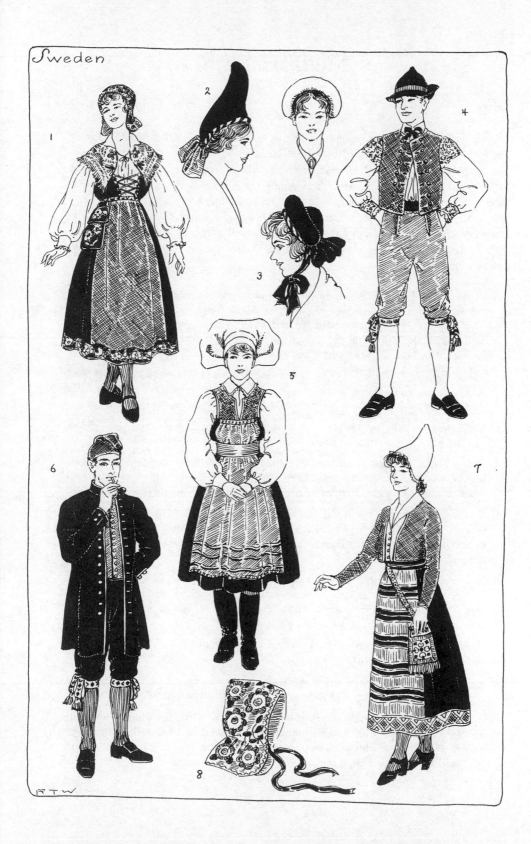

Sweden

❊ Switzerland ❊

Plate 90

see U.S.A. (105)

Switzerland, a federated republic of twenty-two cantons, was the ancient country of Helvetia which was invaded by Julius Caesar in 58 B.C. She obtained her independence from the Holy Roman Empire in 1648. Internal strife took place until 1803 when Napoleon gave Switzerland a new constitution with a president. In sixteen cantons, Swiss-German dialects are spoken by many people and also spoken are French, Italian and Romansh. Concerned with folk-dress disappearing, some Swiss formed a National Costumes League to hold revival gatherings from each canton. They meet for three days, periodically, in regional dress for folk-dancing, singing, alpenhorn concerts and parades.

1. A woman of Fribourg where folk-dress is worn once a month. For bridal and christening affairs, a pincushion hat, neck ruff and fresh-cut flowers pinned to the corselet. The crown of white, with red and black corsage pins above a black velvet band. White blouse with pleated sleeves over gauze. Collarette of French blue lawn, flowered dark blue silk skirt with plain blue apron. Black slippers and stockings.

2. The schlappe, a bonnet of Appenzell Canton. Black and white fan-shaped, pleated gauze wings, white inside, black outside attached to a straw crown. In back, a black ribbon bowknot.

3. A Fribourg wedding headdress. A black bonnet frilled with pink and silver ribbon and the bride's hair braided with black and Roman-striped ribbon.

4. Young woman of Chaffhausen Canton wearing a tiny black velvet calotte and ribbon lappets. Blouse and apron of white linen with black skirt and a green bodice laced and tied with red ribbons. Braided hair with red ribbons, red stockings with red shoes.

5. A farmer from the Canton of Uri in a shepherd's smock of coarse, white linen with a hood. A leather belt and large felt hat often in tricorne style. Cloth or leather breeches in buff color. White, knitted linen thread stockings and shoes with broad tongues and large silver buckles.

6. A woman of Appenzell Canton in a square-cut collar with chains looped from front to back corners. Collar and apron of apricot damask, black velvet laced bodice and dark blue skirt. White linen blouse with ribbon-tied sleeves and apricot silk cap with bowknot in back. White stockings and black slippers.

7. Evolène bride with bonnet of red tulle and Christmas tree balls over a white linen and lace cap with red satin lappets.

8. An everyday bonnet of the Canton of Valais, worn even when farming. Black velvet with red silk crown, beads and rows of narrow black velvet ribbon.

9. A young man of Appenzell in yellow, red and white. White linen shirt and white knitted woolen socks with buckled leather garters. Jacket of Chinese red cloth with yellow and white stitchery. Square, silver buttons and heavy silver fobs. A red scarf and the crossbar braces embroidered in yellow and white. Bright yellow suède breeches and a black felt hat with fresh flowers. Shoes, beige and black.

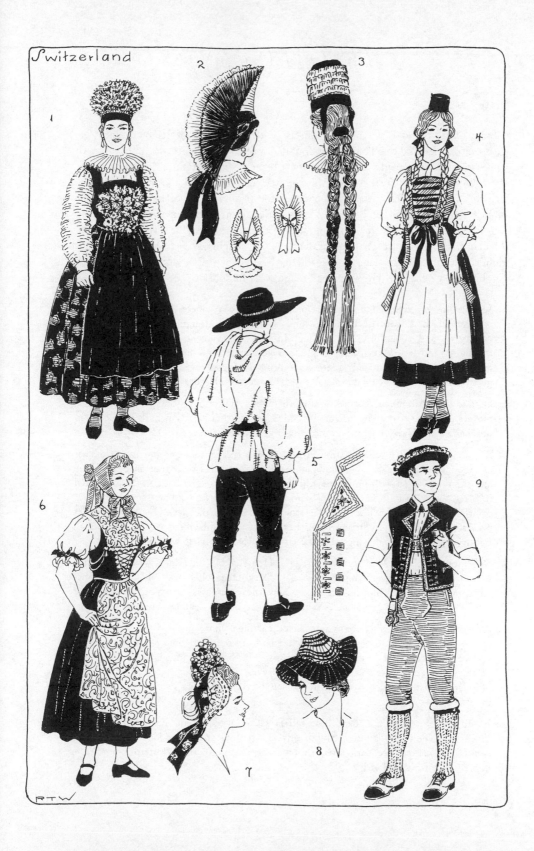

Switzerland

✤ *Thailand (Siam)* ✤

Plate 91

Siam or Thailand is an ancient country with no history of its own until the 12th century. In 1350 the Thai people founded a separate state. In the 15th and 16th centuries it was frequently overrun by the Burmese. In the 16th and 17th centuries the Dutch and Portuguese visited the country and in the 18th century came the British and the French who seized parts of the territory. But Siam was never exploited by colonization. It became a constitutional monarchy in 1932 and during World War II, was seized by Japan. In 1948 Siam changed its English name to Thailand, meaning "free nation." Education is compulsory between the ages of eight and fifteen. The language is Thai, based upon Pali and Sanskrit, with English used officially. The principal religion is Buddhism.

1. A costume gorgeous in fabric and color is that of the Siamese dancer. The skirt or panung which is worn by both men and women, is a straight piece of fabric one yard wide and about three yards long. In this arrangement it is wrapped round the figure and laid into groups of pleats, held secure by a belt. The costume is of red and gold brocade, a red taffeta scarf printed in gold over a bodice of brilliant green taffeta. The pagoda-like metal cap is covered with gilt and sparkling stones.

2. Dressed for a Brahman festival in the regulation uniform of the government employees. A white coat and a bright dark blue panung drawn up in back as shown in number 4. All black, buckled leather shoes and white socks.

3. A young woman of the Miao tribe in blue with sparkling accents and some touches of red. Her dress is dark blue cotton, the apron woven in two lighter shades of blue and the tunic edged with light blue and some silver pieces. The bodice is embroidered in a red zigzag pattern and covered with dangling silver coins. There are two larger coins on the red and white shoulder straps, and round the neck, two silver circlet necklaces, all this display representing her dowry. A crushed red cotton sash and a tightly dressed blue and white checked cotton turban complete the picture.

4. An employee of the Ministry of the Royal Household. White linen or cotton tunic with red and white, self-fringed silk sash. Dark blue collar and cuffs and helmet with gold braid. This illustration shows how the panung is drawn up between the legs in back forming pantaloons. White socks and black leather, buckled shoes.

5. A woman of the Lessu tribe whose silver earrings, hung on a chain, reach from ear to ear. She wears large silver brooches and sewn to her bodice are silver coins and beads. The belt is also sewn with silver. The basic costume is dark blue with green, black and orange banding on the sleeves. The enormous turban, also dark blue, appears to be heavy cording in woolen fabric with strings of beads holding it in place.

6. A villager of Messu in a dark blue taffeta jacket wadded and lined with Chinese green silk. The jacket is fastened with tiny ball buttons and fabric loops. His panung is probably cotton, also dark blue, and the carryall, or in our Western usage "tote bag," is red with gold stripes.

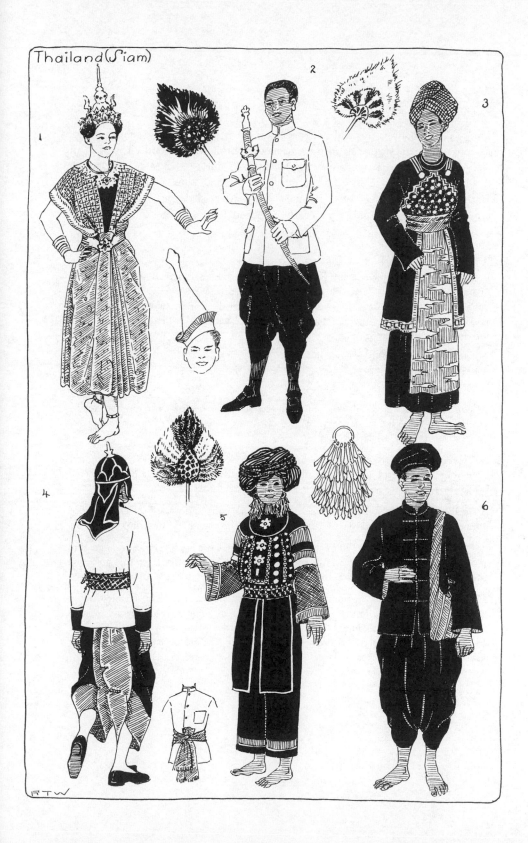

Thailand (Siam)

❈ *Tibet* ❈

Plate 92

Tibet is nominally a dependency of China in Asia with its capital, Lhasa, situated on the highest plateau in the world. Buddhism was introduced in the 7th century A.D. China first took over control in 1720 during the Manchu Dynasty and until the late 19th century, the country was generally closed to foreigners. In 1959, the Tibetan revolt against Communist rule was crushed, the Dalai Lama fleeing to India. The Communists placed the Panchen Lama on the Tibetan throne. Lamaism is the religion, a form of Buddhism.

1. A bride in ceremonial dress with beauty spots on her forehead. The basic gown is of flowered black velvet with panels of velvet and Roman-striped silk and strings of beads hanging over a red silk skirt. A collarette of flowered yellow silk, pink silk cuffs and a red scarf round the upper arms fastened with turquoise jewelry. Her peaked velvet headdress, which hangs down the back, has an ivory crescent with red balls and the hair ornaments are turquoise.

2. An aristocrat, as is evident from the long sleeves covering his hands which he need not use to gain a living. He wears a yellow silk brocade robe with a gold and red hat topped with a tassel. His white felt boots have peaked-toes.

3. A lama of the reformed Tibetan Church in ceremonial robes of dark red and yellow woolen cloth with the tufted felt hat. He of the celibate yellow hat may not marry but a man of the red hat sect may.

4. A Tibetan lama in a rich yellow satin robe with a jacket of yellow satin brocade. The front panel of the decorative yellow hat is outlined with gilt braid and his felt boots are fur-lined.

5. A small boy in a dark blue cloth robe with blue silk cuffs and a cord sash. A wadded jumper of deep yellow velvet and dark blue felt boots with white trim.

6. A little girl in a wadded, yellow velvet, smock-like blouse with a wide orange sash and blue velvet cuffs. The very full skirt is of bright blue cotton. Her cap gives the effect of a tam-o'-shanter with red and white balls for decor and she also wears earrings.

7. The mother of the child in number 6 in the same style of dress. The wadded upper section is of violet silk brocade sleeved and sashed in orange, the sleeves brocaded and the sash plain silk. The full skirt, like the little girl's, is of cotton but in a brilliant blue-green. Her coif is dressed in pompadour fashion, probably over a frame, with an effective headdress of large brown and yellow amber beads.

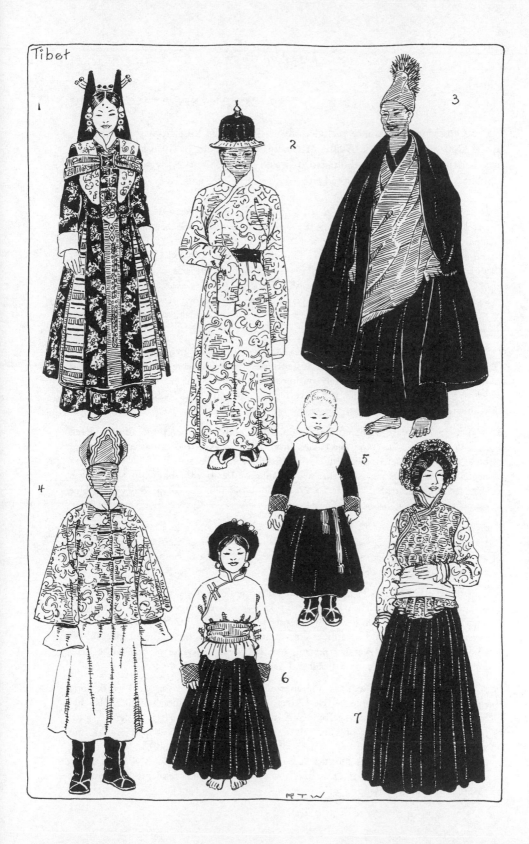

Tibet

1

2

3

4

5

6

7

RTW

❧ *Turkey* ❧

Plate 93   see ALBANIA, ANATOLIA, IRAQ

The Ottoman Empire once included all of the Middle East from the Black Sea to the Gulf of Aden. After 1700 it gradually declined and by 1918 so much territory had been lost that the Sultanate fell and in 1925 Turkey was proclaimed a republic. The costumes illustrated are of the late 19th and early 20th centuries.

1. A Moslem woman of Salonika in street dress until it was decreed in 1928 that the enveloping and concealing costume be banned. She wears the babouche, the peak-toed, heelless slipper of fabric or soft leather, and the chalwar, full pantaloons to the ankles. Over the pantaloons, an embroidered chemise or blouse, an entari, belted with handsome fabric or jeweled girdle. Then a long, sleeveless, embroidered coat of silk or velvet, the caftan. The yashmak or face veil was of sheer voile, two squares folded diagonally, the folds placed above and below eyes and falling over shoulders and bosom. And lastly, the feridgé or woman's cloak, a heavy, voluminous manteau with cape in back.

2. A Turkish-Albanian soldier in a uniform of white linen and green woolen cloth with green embroidery. A softly pleated fustanella is worn over a green cloth skirt and the green sleeves are slashed. The fur piece backed with felt has many uses. A red felt fez with gold tassel and red, peak-toed shoes with small gold pompons worn with green woolen stockings.

3. A Turkish-Albanian woman with flowing hair and a rich costume. Embroidered chemise of white silk crêpe, the entari, over which is worn the caftan of robin's-egg blue satin embroidered with gilt and belted in multi-colored silk. The outer cloak or feridgé is of lacquer-red velvet with hanging sleeves of robin's-egg blue velvet. All pieces including the red felt fez are gilt embroidered, the fez graced with a blue tassel. On her feet, babouches of red velvet.

4. A Moslem woman in village costume. Over a fold of white lace on her head, she wears an embroidered, rose-colored cotton shawl. Her dress consists of two pieces, a sleeveless chemise over an ankle-length, straight-leg chalwar, both garments of pink and white striped cotton.

5. Christian-Turkish Bulgarians adopted the full pantaloons for "at home" dress, here in changeable green taffeta over white stockings and red moroccan leather slippers. The chemise of sheer white voile has flaring wrist ruffles, silver buttons and a heavy silver belt. The rose-colored silk caftan, quilted-lined, has ribbed green silk sleeves embroidered in black. Over her flowing hair she wears a square of fine white linen folded and kept in place by a headband of red silk over silver galon.

6. A merchant of Yemen wearing the masculine dolama, an outer cloak with long sleeves, shown here in blue velvet. Under it he wears the djubbeh which also has long sleeves, is open down the front and is fur-lined in winter. It is of heavy, gray-blue silk. Under the vest of blue velvet, a shirt or mintan of striped orange and white crêpe, and over the vest, a sash of striped silk. His headdress is interesting because he has draped his blue-tasseled red fez with white cloth. Modern Turkish men have adopted Western dress and today, the masculine fez and the feminine yashmak has all but disappeared.

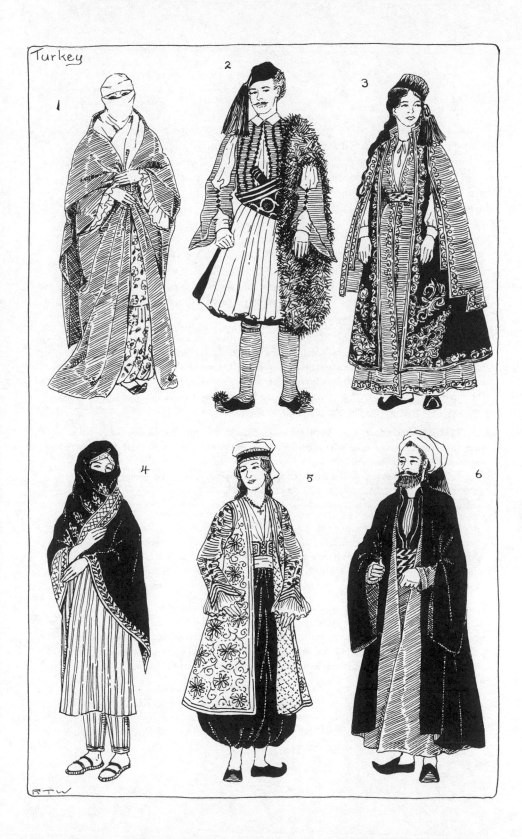

Turkey

1

2

3

4

5

6

RTW

❊ *Tyrol* ❊

Plate 94   see AUSTRIA, GERMANY, ITALY

Tyrol, a province of western Austria, is situated in the Alps and also borders on Germany, Switzerland and Italy. It was inhabited in early times by the Celtic race and at one period was part of the Roman Empire. It passed into the hands of Austria in 1363. It was ceded to Bavaria by Napoleon in 1805 and reunited with Austria in 1814 after the revolt against Napoleon. In 1919 the southern part was transferred to Italy and in 1939, after disturbances among the populace, the borders were again revised.

1. An Austrian woman of the Otz Valley in a laced black velvet bodice over a white muslin blouse and a flowered silk neckerchief. The black cotton skirt is partially covered by a gayly printed silk apron with the apron strings brought round and tied in front. Her beige felt hat is decked with plumage, her socks are red and her slippers, black.

2. A Venetian symphony of color. The breeches are brown velvet or suède leather with tan cording. The tapestry embroidery on the brown velvet belt is executed in varied tones of brown. A white shirt with a stubby red silk scarf and a waistcoat of lacquer red cloth finished with yellow braid. The crossbar braces are pea green leather and the felt hat of the same green with brown and white feathers. All buttons are ivory-colored, the same color for the stockings worn with brown slippers.

3. An Italian fête costume worn on Corpus Christi Day. A white blouse with frilled lace collar and sleeves and a red bodice combined with green silk and laced with yellow ribbon. The crown-like headdress is fashioned of black velvet with a tall, pointed top of iridescent silk sewn with gilt and crystal beads. An onyx cross hangs on a coral bead necklace. White stockings and black slippers.

4. An Austrian in Tyrolese gala dress with breeches of black leather or cloth made festive with tan cording and red leg ties. A slate gray cloth jacket with peacock green cloth cuffs and embroidered tabs of the same color. The wide belt is black, embroidered in varied brown tones, with crossbar braces matching. His shirt is white and the short ends are one red and one green. The black felt hat mounts a dashing feather, along with white woolen socks and black leather shoes.

5. A Bavarian "mountain maid" carrying her small keg of brandy to revive the energy of weary climbers. A brandy goblet in her hand and a blue and white napkin tucked into her belt. She wears a laced black velvet bodice over a white cotton blouse and a pale silk fringed shawl. The skirt and the apron are pink. The tall-crowned, black felt hat is ornamented with flowers and pink cord with tassel. The slippers are black with white stockings.

6. A Bavarian mountain guide in leather dress and rope. His jacket is copper-colored and his breeches of a much darker hue. Brown, too, is the jaunty cap with feather panache. The waistcoat is leather but in dark green, the knitted woolen socks are stone gray and his leather shoes, black.

Tyrol

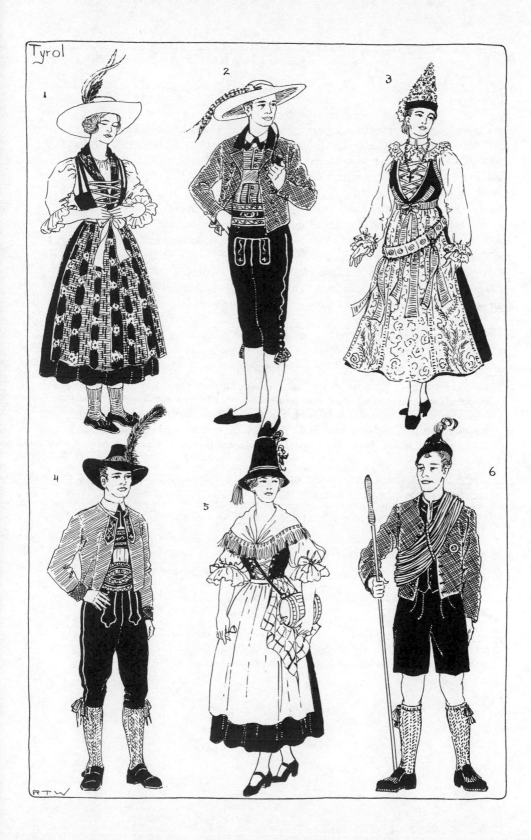

❊ U.S.A. Alaska ❊

Plate 95

Known originally as Russian Alaska because first discovered by Russian voyagers in 1741. Claimed by Russia, the land was sold to the United States in 1867 for $7,200,000. Territorial status was established in 1912 and in 1958, Alaska became our forty-ninth state. Discoveries of rich gold fields occurred in 1896. Unearthed small tools indicate occupation of Alaska as far back as 2500 B.C. It appears that the original people came from Asia by way of Bering Strait, many moving south to warmer climate. Those that settled in the Arctic region became known as Eskimos, a word meaning "those who eat raw flesh." Eskimos, Indians and Aleuts make up about a sixth of the population with scattered white settlers. When under Russian control, Greek Catholic missionaries brought Christianity to the natives so that most belong to some Christian sect. The natives speak their own respective languages. Public schools are supervised by the U.S. Government.

1. Totem pole, carved and painted and usually attached to the front of the house. Ornamented with mystic, symbolic signs.

2. Woman carrying her baby in the hood of the parka. Tunic, shirt and breeches of sealskin with the fur to the inside. Tunic ornamented with red woolen bands appliquéd with green and white leather motifs and edged with dog fur. White leather leggings. Red leather boots with appliqué as above. Sealskin cap with fabric trimming. Of the 1870's, such an outfit made by the wearer would require a year's work along with her other chores and no sewing machine available.

3. Modern navy blue parka with fur-edged hood is worn over the accompanying fur parka and breeches. Rickrack braid trimming. Red leather boots, fur-topped and appliquéd with red on white leather.

4. Woven rug of colored wools with slashed leather fringe.

5. Little girl in fur boots, shirt and tunic and a modern overdress or parka of brightly printed calico with attached fur-edged hood.

6. Man's outfit of fox or wolf fur. Slashed leather fringe, sandals and thongs.

7. A baby in white bear parka and hood. Mittens and leggings of skin with the fur side in.

8. Man's costume of the 1870's of sealskin with fur side in. Red and yellow knitted wool trimming. Mittens fashioned of bear's claws with the claws attached. Fur-lined brown leather boots edged with dog's fur and trimmed with yellow leather.

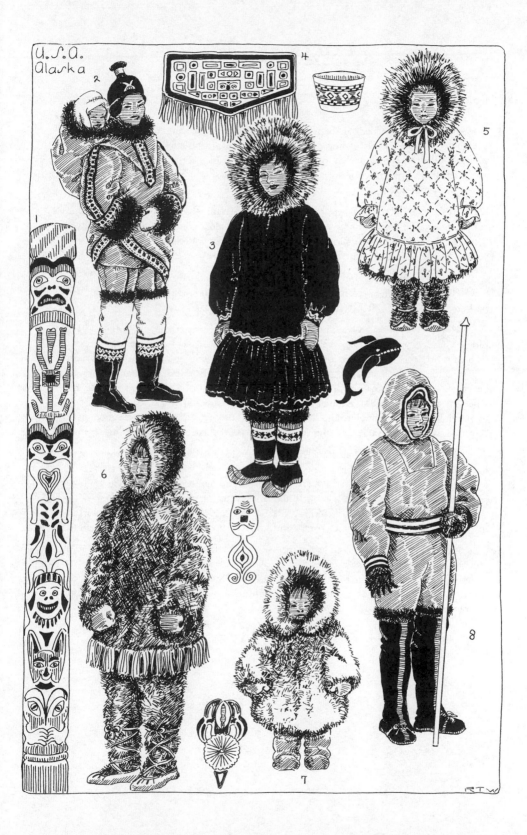

U.S.A.
Alaska

✣ U.S.A. Cowboy ✣

Plate 96

1. A western "dude rancher" in batwing cowhide chaparajos, commonly called chaps, over blue or brown pants of heavy cotton. The chaps are fastened in back by leather thongs pulled through conchas of nickel or silver which provide decoration down the side of the leg. Brown leather belt, boots and spurs, white cotton shirt and a felt or straw sombrero.

2. Here, we come full cycle from the embroidered peasant costume of Europe to this 20th century California riding outfit. A white silk blouse, dark blue cotton velvet bolero and pants, the three pieces embroidered in a floral design of green, rose and yellow. A hat of felt or straw in white or black.

3. A California habit which reveals its Spanish-Mexican influence. Braid-bound, black velvet bolero with putty-colored whipcord breeches. White cotton shirt with red silk neckerchief. A black felt hat and black leather boots, belt and holster.

4. A cowboy of Montana, Wyoming or the Dakotas wearing chaps of Angora goat hide. Those of sheepskin are called woollies. A woolen vest or "weskit" over a woolen shirt, the leather cartridge belt with accompanying gun, leather boots and a gay cotton or silk bandana knotted round the neck. His Mexican sombrero might be beige, white, black or brown felt. The sombrero came to be known as the Stetson when in the early 1870's, a Philadelphia hat-maker named John B. Stetson decided to put his effort into producing a quality hat for the cowboy. The "ten-gallon hat" acquired world-wide fame and, for most cowboys, the hat lasted a lifetime.

5. A typical western outfit consisting of red and blue plaided gingham blouse and dark blue denim pants. A black felt hat of Spanish style with chin-strap and black leather boots with tan leather tracery. Those strong cotton pants known as blue jeans or Levis are more than a century old and were the creation of a Levi Strauss who went to California in 1850 seeking his fortune which he found not in gold but in his idea of indigo blue denim pants reinforced with copper rivets at crucial points.

6. Chaparajos or "California leggings" of deerskin with the hair left on the front and outer sides for warmth and protection from moisture. They are suspended by a tooled leather belt laced in front. Tanned leather without the hair is used for work dress. A western shirt of gabardine with contrasting-colored piping and a bright colored bandana. Felt hat, leather boots and gun.

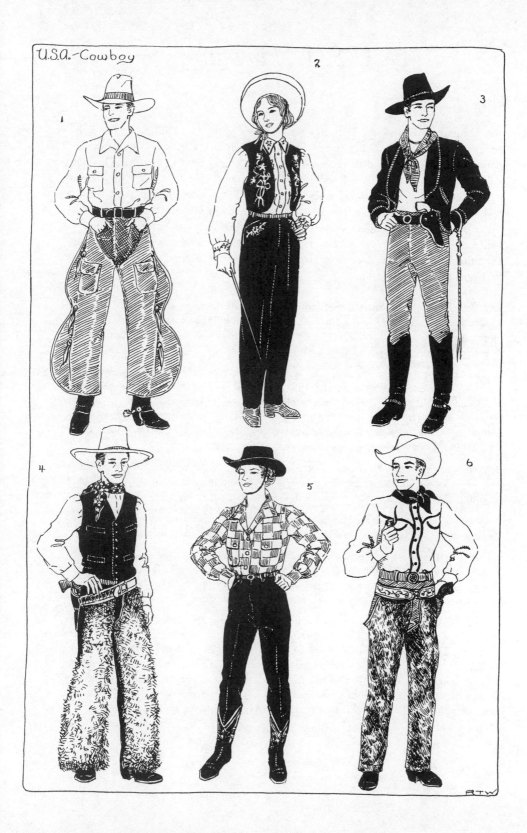

U.S.A. - Cowboy

✶ U.S.A. Hawaii ✶

Plate 97

According to legend the islands were first settled by a small group of Polynesians about 500 B.C. Other immigrants arrived in the 12th and 13th centuries. American whalers reached there in the early 19th century and American Christian missionaries in 1820. Today, Buddhism is the strongest Eastern faith in Hawaii with several of its numerous branches represented. The United States, Great Britain and France recognized the independence of the Islands in 1844. In 1875, a reciprocity treaty with the United States was secured and in 1894, Hawaii became a republic. It became United States territory in 1900 and in 1960, became our fiftieth state. An educational note is that more than 11,000 students enroll annually at the university in Honolulu.

1. A Hawaiian-born Japanese in her native dress. A silk kimono of white and sapphire blue printed with motifs of red and light hues of blue. The red silk obi has a design printed in yellow and a white silk under-kimono shows at the neck. White padded cotton tabi are worn with yellow zori with red straps.

2. The traditional formal dress of the upper class Filipino, Hawaiian born, bears the stamp of Western fashions of the 19th century at the time the islands became a republic. This gown is taken from a photograph of the late 1930's and is of Nile green gauze striped in white. The starched, sheer fabric is rengue made from native pineapple. The crisp double fichu or pañuelo and the bodice or camisa are ornamented with purple velvet flowers, also reminiscent of the mauve decade.

3. A formal version of the simple muu-muu, the shift that American college girls discovered in the 1950's and brought home to wear. Our illustration of the printed pink cotton dress is of the late 1930's, and the wearer is a "Hawaiian-born Hawaiian".

4. A young Chinese woman, Hawaiian-born, in her native cheongsam of Venetian red satin combined with gold colored satin and brown embroidery. Brown silk slippers.

5. The Hula dance was the classic Hawaiian dance so frankly based upon all phases of life that the early missionaries were prompted to suppress it. Revived in modern times the performance dwells instead upon the gaieties of life. The dancer is in bare feet, wearing a skirt of rich green ti-leaves, a bodice and embroidered silk and flower leis.

6. A Hawaiian-born Korean woman in her national dress, this of dark blue and white although in Korea white cotton is traditionally for everyday wear and principally for adults. The skirt pleated to a bosom band is snugly fastened round under the armpits and a blouse or vest put on next. Over the latter goes a short bolero tied with a one-loop bowknot fastening left to right. Western dress has been generally adopted by men for formal use and traveling, but for everyday and sportswear, men, boys and male visitors, all wear slacks, shorts and the gaudy Hawaiian aloha shirts.

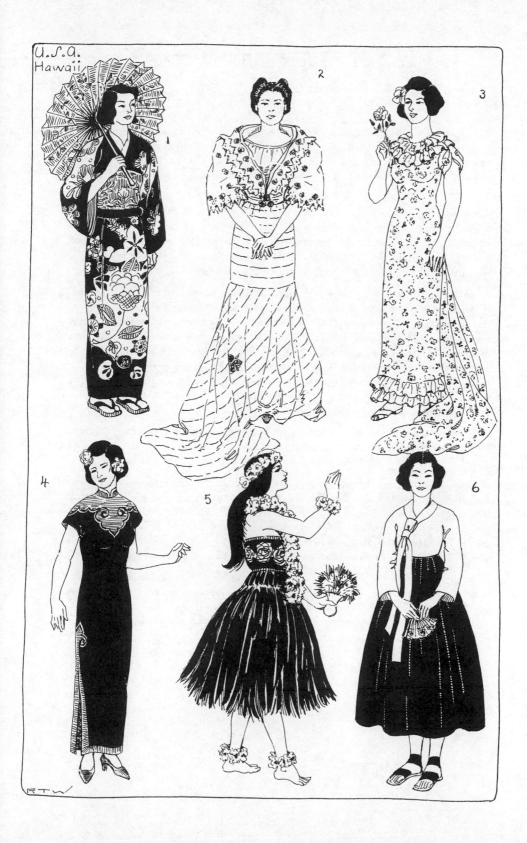

U.S.A.
Hawaii

✻ U.S.A. Here and There ✻

Plate 98

1. A member of the Russian Colony called "The Old Believers" whose ancestors seceded from the 17th century Russian Church and settled in Erie, Pennsylvania, in the 1890's. Our balalaika player is garbed in a green silk smock with hand embroidery and belted with a hand-loomed sash. His breeches are tan woolen cloth and his leather boots are black.

2. A Queen of Laurel Blossoms is crowned and fêted annually in Stroudsburg, Pennsylvania, to celebrate that event of great beauty. It is typical of the spring festivals in honor of native blooms held throughout the country. This royal costume is of lace dyed pale blue with a plum-colored robe embroidered with a gold border and edged with white fur. On her head, a tiara of simulated jewels.

3. From Poland in the 1880's came a group of refugees to our shores. Being farmers, they settled on some acres of virgin, moist black land in Orange County, New York, and proceeded to grow onions in the perfect soil. Success finally crowned their efforts and they named their new home "Black Acres". Each year since 1938 they have celebrated the harvest in song and dance, wearing Polish festival costumes. Over a white cotton shirt with a red silk tie is worn a sleeveless jacket of either red or blue cloth, a red sash and white cotton breeches striped with red. A square cap is banded in black of either fur or velvet and ornamented with, of course, an onion plant as a panache from which float colored ribbons.

4. A young woman of the Russian colony in Erie, Pennsylvania, noted in number 1. Hers is a white voile blouse, a red cotton skirt with a hand-loomed sash. Her head shawl is white silk fringed and printed in brown. White stockings and black slippers.

5. A Buddhist priest, member of a company of Kalmuks, the descendants of some ancient Buddhist Mongolian tribes who escaped the armies of Genghis Khan by fleeing to the Lower Volga. These very recently arrived immigrants settled in Freewood Acres, New Jersey, where they worship in a small temple, a garage-like building of cinder block but with a colorful, religiously decorated interior. The lama is robed in saffron and red, his saffron bonnet lined with red and in his hands, his prayer beads.

6. A young woman of the Polish colony noted in number 3. Her festival costume consists of a lace-trimmed white batiste blouse and apron, a flowered cotton skirt, a black velvet corselet with inserts of green silk and laced with red ribbons. Black slippers with white stockings and a wreath of flowers upon her head.

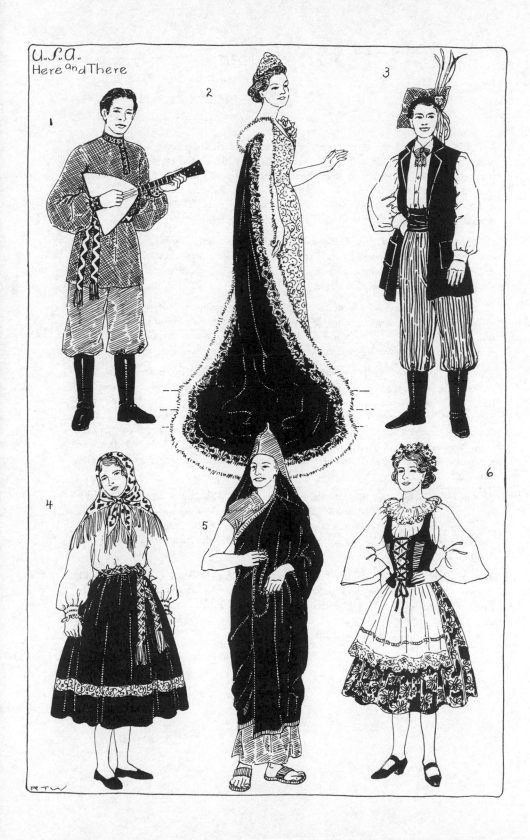

U.S.A.
Here and There

1

2

3

4

5

6

R.T.W.

❧ *U.S.A. Indian* ❧

Plate 99

see NEW MEXICO AND TEXAS,
OREGON AND WYOMING

1. A Blackfoot chief of the 19th century, the dressiest of all the tribes. Their garments were beautifully made of skillfully tanned skins. His black moccasins were elaborate with embroidery of beads and brightly colored porcupine quills. A tunic of natural colored deerskin with leggings of a deep gold color. Bands of embroidery of bead and porcupine work, fringed with thinned-out scalp locks. The pipe is of steatite, wound with bead and quill work and further decorated with a few scalp locks.

2. Contemporary Seminole dress fashioned of cotton stripes sewn together on a portable sewing machine. The upper section is royal blue, the skirt a deep pink with alternating strips of yellow, black, sky blue and white. The hair is dressed in pompadour style reminiscent of the Gibson Girl days.

3. "Red Jacket", Seneca chief and orator, 1758(?)–1830, wearing the red jacket presented to him by an English officer and the silver medal, a gift of Washington. The coat was trimmed with silver braid and bead fringe and tied with a handsome silk sash. A fur cap and deerskin leggings and moccasins.

4. The Indians of Zuni in New Mexico retain a decided Spanish influence in their pottery and jewelry design. They specialize in turquoise, all the pieces shown on numbers 4 and 6 being turquoise. The costume is of homespun black cloth with blouse and belt of green or red silk. The underskirt is gayly printed cotton and the deerskin leggings and soft low boots are white deerskin. On her head an olla, she being an "olla bearer", a common sight. The olla is a round pot of baked clay with a wide mouth in which is cooked olla, a meat and vegetable dish highly seasoned and minced.

5. A Mohawk chief of the late 18th century wearing a white linen smock with silver armlets. A red woolen blanket, black leather leggings and white, beaded deerskin moccasins. He wears a leather baldric, his pipe and leather tobacco pouch on a beaded chain and a locket on a silver chain. A single, slim feather is held by the scalp lock.

6. Zuni women of the Pueblo Land have worn the same frock of hand-woven black cloth since pre-Columbian days, but the native silver and turquoise are modern. The dress is belted with red cloth embroidered in yellow and a narrow green and red line finished with two turquoise brooches ornamenting the skirt. The leggings and soft low boots are of white deerskin.

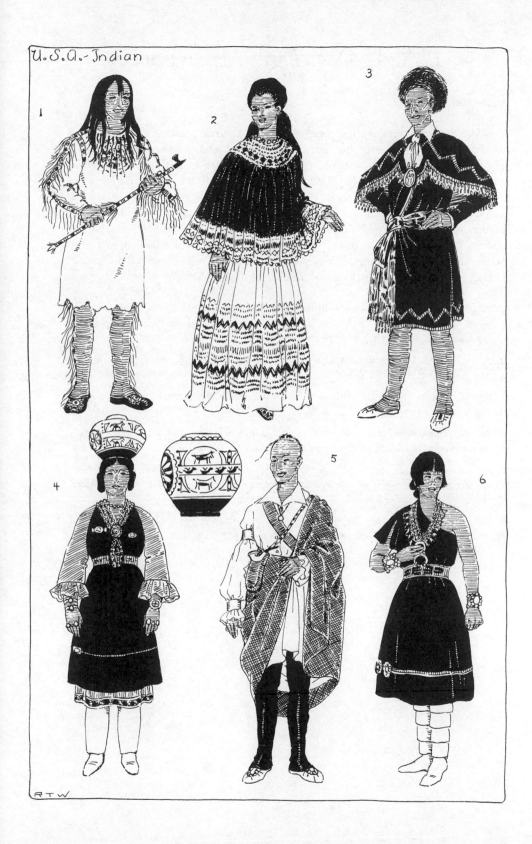

U.S.A.-Indian

✳ U.S.A. Natchez, Mississippi ✳

Plate 100

While these costumes are not regional dress in the real sense of the term, they are remembered pictures of the ante-bellum days of Old Natchez in Mississippi during that era of great wealth and fabulous mansions. For nearly a century since the War Between the States, Natchez barely survived, but today things have changed for the better with wealth again returning by way of industrial plants and oil instead of cotton. Many of the palatial homes have been restored to much of their former beauty and since 1932, have been opened as museums to paying visitors. On these festive occasions the ladies wear the beautiful crinoline gowns of yesteryear that their ancestors, in many cases, bought in Paris. Thousands of people attend the openings held each year during "Pilgrimage Month".

1. A gown of pale blue cashmere ornamented with picot-edged lavender satin. Sheer white lawn undersleeves. A bonnet of black taffeta with pink and black striped ribbons and the face framed with pink roses.

2. A young miss in a cotton frock, white striped with blue and red over a crinoline and frilled white muslin pantalets.

3. Sports or summer masculine dress in natural colored linen, striped cotton trousers and a straw hat.

4. A young man in a black velvet bolero over a fine white muslin shirt. His trousers are of brown and black plaided woolen cloth and his black shoes have beige uppers.

5. A morning negligee composed of an outer and an underdress of white cambric with fluted ruffles. The cap is of fine muslin with lace-edged lappets and a striped colored ribbon tied round the crown.

6. An evening gown of robin's-egg blue peau de soie flounced with blonde lace headed with guimpe. Bowknots of velvet ribbon of a deeper blue. The cap of white tulle and blue ribbon has pink roses set in tulle rosettes.

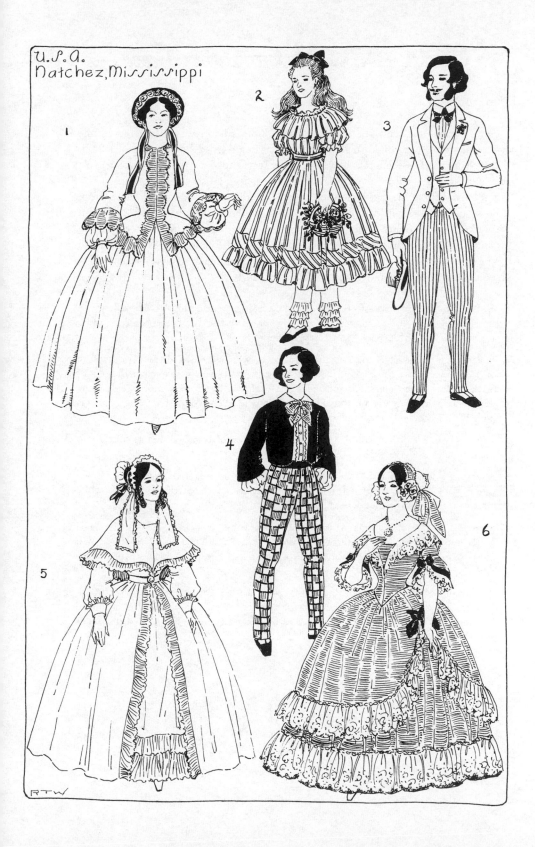

U.S.A.
Natchez, Mississippi

1

2

3

4

5

6

RTW

❋ U.S.A. New Mexico and Texas ❋

Plate 101

New Mexico, originally the country of the Zuni Indians, was discovered by the Spaniards in 1530, explored in the 1540's and was governed by Mexico after 1821. Included in the Gadsden Purchase of 1853, it was ceded to the United States in 1848 and in 1912, became the forty-seventh state admitted to the Union.

The discovery and exploration of Texas by the Spaniards took place from 1519 to 1684 and occupation by the Spaniards in 1715. By treaty with Spain in 1819, the United States' claim to Texas was relinquished, Texas becoming a province of Mexico. Seeking annexation to the United States, Texas was admitted to the Union in 1845 and after the settlement of boundary disputes followed by secession, she was re-admitted to the Union in 1870.

1. A San Antonian in his festival garb. Of black velvet with a full-sleeved, yellow silk shirt and a luxurious red silk scarf. His faja or wide belt is of pleated black satin, a black felt hat, white socks and black leather pumps.

2. A Pueblo Indian woman of Zuni, New Mexico, whose style of dress dates back to pre-Columbian days. The pointed-bodice bib and skirt which have always been of black or dark blue homespun, and the white buckskin boots are centuries old. Here, the bodice-point is black and the skirt blue with a belt of dark red. The blouse is pink with black polka-dots and the shawl, white.

3. A young woman of San Antonio in her festival gown of beruffled orange taffeta and hibiscus flowers in her hair.

4. A young Pueblo Indian woman whose pointed-bib dress is red and white striped cotton with a green hem and red belt. She wears a white fringed shawl, white buckskin boots and carries a black pottery water jug.

5. A glittering festival costume worn during San Jacinto week in San Antonio. The white muslin is beaded and threaded with black velvet ribbon. A skirt of red and green satin is sewn with sparkling paillettes and jet. The pleated, fan-shaped head-dress is of white muslin.

6. A Navajo Indian of New Mexico wearing an artistic costume consisting of dark gray trousers, a smock of deep purple velveteen and a gray silk sash. His headband is orange silk and the necklace, buttons and bracelets are silver. His beaded moccasins are white buckskin.

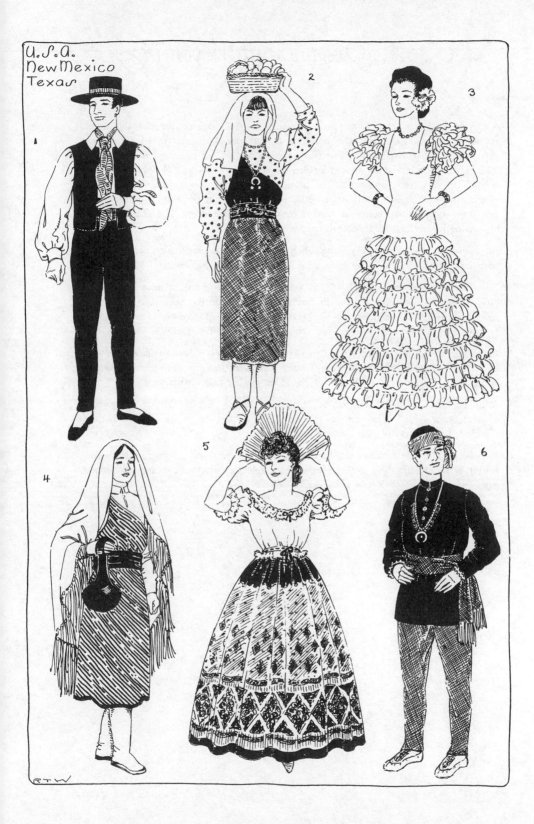

U.S.A.
New Mexico
Texas

1

2

3

4

5

6

RTW

✳ *U.S.A. Oregon and Wyoming* ✳

Plate 102

1. A Cayuse Indian queen in a handsomely beaded festival costume worn for the annual round-up held in Pendleton, Oregon. It is of soft deerskin, self-fringed. The upper cape-like section is dyed a turquoise blue with motifs beaded in white, red and black. The wrap-around skirt is natural golden beige. Her boots are of white buckskin beaded in black, red and brown. The beaded headband is white with red and black motifs and the hair is braided and lengthened with strips of deerskin and animal fur. An eagle feather and a couple of flowers complete the headdress. The skirt is secured by a wide leather belt studded with copper ornaments.

2. An accordion player on a Wyoming ranch in a dark blue cloth shirt, beige breeches with leather belt, a brown felt with a brick-red silk band and boots of black leather.

3. To southeastern Oregon in the 1890's came the Basques of the Spanish Pyrenees to raise sheep. This young woman in her black lace mantilla worn for the annual fiesta, has definitely retained the airs and graces of her forebears. Her dress is of yellow silk with pleated flounces, her slippers black and her stockings white.

4. A "cowgirl" or female bronco rider of the Wild West Show held annually at Lander, Wyoming. Her outfit consists of black breeches, an orange suède jacket, white shirt, black scarf and black felt hat. Her leather boots are also black.

5. A queen of an annual floral parade held in Portland, Oregon. The filmy gown is of white tulle with a white fur collar. She wears a sparkling diadem and her hands are gloved in white lace mitts.

6. A bronco rider of the Show in Lander, Wyoming. A plaid gingham shirt accompanies pants of light blue denim plus a black felt sombrero, a brilliant silk neckerchief, brown leather belt and black leather boots.

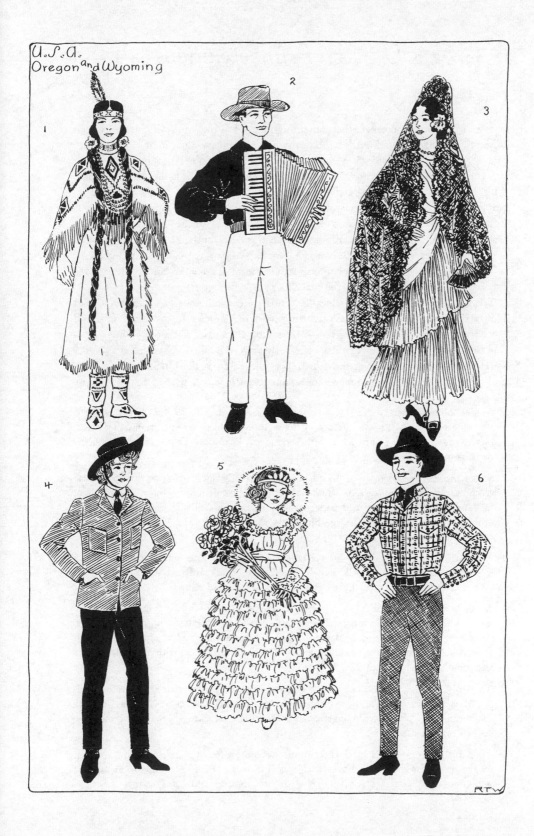

U.S.A.
Oregon and Wyoming

❊ U.S.A. Pennsylvania ❊

Plate 103

The Mennonites, one of the denominations of Protestant Christians which originated in Switzerland, settled in Germantown, Pennsylvania, in 1683. There are many sects of the Christian Mennonites or "Plain People", mostly of German descent. The most unswerving from ancient customs and beliefs is the Amish branch. The men dress in black, they eschew any ornamentation such as lapels and buttons, using instead, hooks and eyes and strings as fasteners. Buttons appear to be permitted on the everyday workshirt which might be gray, beige or gray-blue. Men wear their hair cut in Dutch fashion with bangs, the mustache is forbidden, and every male after marriage must wear a beard. Women wear black in public or solid muted colors but may don a printed frock at home. A dainty white lawn cap is worn indoors and under the black bonnet when going out.

The Quakers, who call themselves "Friends", are a religious sect founded about 1650, who wished to purify the Church in advocating simpler forms of worship and daily living. Because they were given to trembling under the stress of religious emotion or when questioned about their beliefs, they were dubbed "Quakers".

The Shaker sect which was formed in 1747 differs from the Quakers in doctrine and practice. The name originated in a dance which was a part of their worship.

1. A Mennonite woman in gray with bonnet and jacket of a darker hue than her skirt, of homespun cotton or wool according to season. A black kerchief round her neck, black cotton stockings and black leather oxfords. The straw basket is no doubt her own handiwork.

2. Shaker dress is most simple in design but not so totally unchanging as the Mennonite costume. There was much more choice of color in the soft tones of blue, gray, brown, tan and white, and pin-striped patterns were worn. This Shaker youth is in brown or blue woolen cloth with a large black hat of beaver felt. He wears calfskin shoes with knitted blue or gray stockings.

3. A typical Quaker costume of brown taffeta with folded fine white kerchief tucked into the belt and a white silk shawl. The bonnet is of stiffened white lawn worn over a frilled lace cap and the reticule is of white corded silk.

4. A Shaker costume of the late 18th century of tan alpaca with the kerchief of sheer white lawn. The underbodice is also white lawn with pointed collar tabs. Over her arm, a three-quarter length cape of natural colored homespun linen with a deep collar. The severe-looking bonnet is of brown percale with a pleated ruffle and small ties under the chin.

5. An Amish woman in her long, black woolen cape, a garment that dates from medieval days and was worn all over Europe. Under the black bonnet with pleated flounce she wears the "always-worn-lingerie-cap". Her black stockings are ribbed and the leather oxfords are black.

6. An Amish farmer in his black, homespun woolen jacket, waistcoat and trousers, all the garments fastened with hooks and eyes. He wears a white cotton or linen shirt with fold-over collar, a black felt hat with ribbon band and black leather shoes.

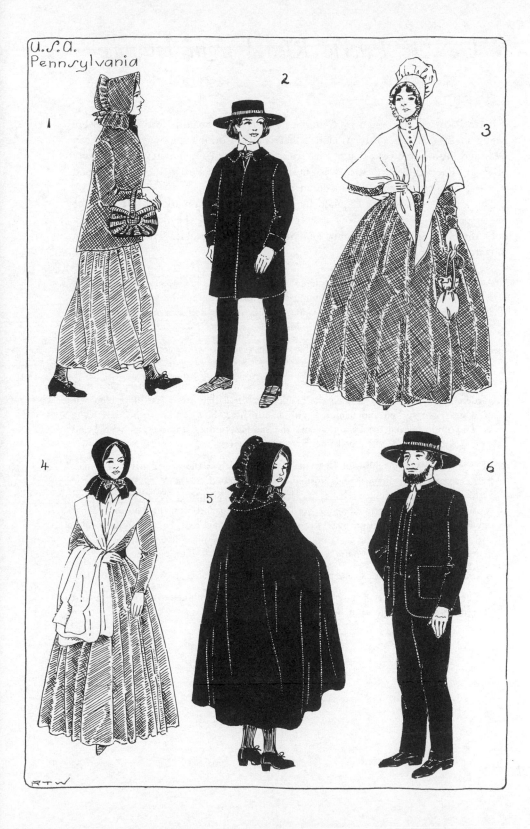

U.S.a.
Pennsylvania

1

2

3

4

5

6

RTW

❧ U.S.A. Puerto Rico-Virgin Islands ❧

Plate 104

Porto Rico was discovered by Columbus in 1493 and Spanish fortifications were begun in 1533. American troops landed there in 1898 during the Spanish-American War and in the same year, Puerto Rico was ceded to the United States by the Treaty of Paris. The name Porto Rico was officially changed to Puerto Rico in 1932 and in 1948, the governorship was made an elective office.

The Virgin Islands were acquired by purchase from Denmark in 1916–1917 for use as a naval base forming our eastern-most outpost. Of the fifty small islands, only three, St. Thomas, St. John, and St. Croix, are sizeable. They were given universal suffrage in 1938.

1. A native of St. Thomas who no doubt made everything she wears, the straw hat with black ribbon band, her blue and white striped cotton dress and the cotton apron of blue print on white. Her sandals could also be her own manufacture. Her marketing bag is a simple length of folded canvas.

2. A Puerto Rican drummer in dark blue cotton trousers, white cotton shirt, colored silk neckerchief and fringed straw hat.

3. A native of St. Thomas selling fruits, vegetables and flowers, probably from her own garden. She carries her wares on the padded crown of her straw hat. The blouse is of white lawn tucked and trimmed with handmade white cotton crochet lace. The skirt of multi-colored striped cotton and the sandals, simply leather soles with braid straps. Around her neck a polka-dotted cotton square.

4. In French Village, a suburb of Charlotte Amalie which is the capital of St. Thomas, live descendants of Bretons and Normans who migrated to the West Indies in the 17th century. The women create gay hats of braided palm-leaf splits, dyed and sewn into smart, exaggerated styles worn by both men and women. The second hat down with mourning band was worn by a man. The first hat is natural color and reddish-brown, the third, natural color with a blue silk ribbon and the fourth, a deep bluish-purple with natural-colored crown and dark blue anchor.

5. A small native of St. Croix and her goat. She wears a printed frock and a straw hat.

6. A Puerto Rican dancer in a white taffeta frilled skirt combined with a bodice and draped apron of orange satin. Gold sandals.

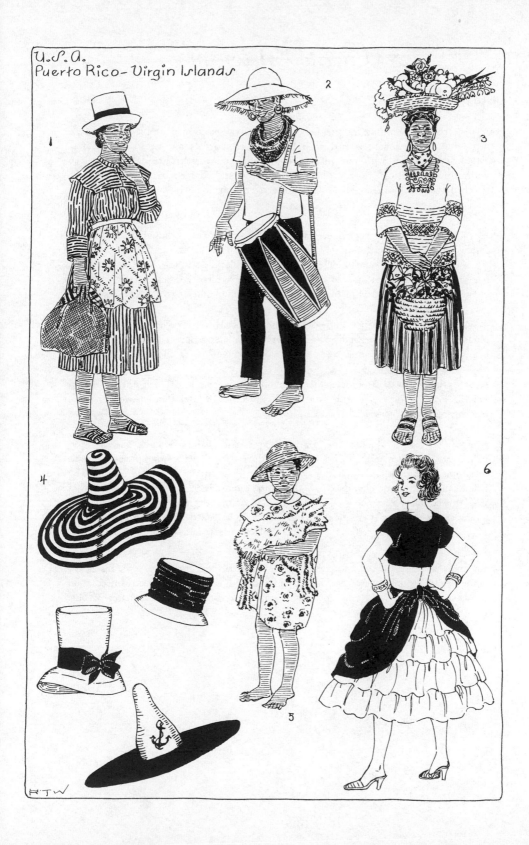

U.S.A.
Puerto Rico - Virgin Islands

❊ U.S.A. Wisconsin ❊

Plate 105

1. A dancer's Swiss costume of the Labor Day festival performed at New Glarus. A soft white cotton blouse is tied with black velvet wristlets and worn with a red cotton skirt banded with gilt ribbon. The apron and corselet are of black velvet with simulated lacings of gilt ribbon on the corselet. The bonnet is fashioned of starched white frills mounted on a black velvet crown and white lappets floating in back. Black slippers and white stockings.

2. A young Scandinavian performer, member of the Norway, Denmark and Iceland colony on Washington Island on Lake Michigan. Her blouse and apron are fine white linen, the apron embroidered in red. The black cloth skirt and a red cloth bolero are embroidered in red and yellow. She wears the Scandinavian square bonnet of red cloth tied with black velvet ribbons. Red stockings and black slippers.

3. A young woman in Swiss festival costume of black velvet with white organdie blouse and a sky-blue organdie apron. Her corn-colored straw hat is turned up at one side and held by a pink rose. White stockings and black slippers.

4. A Swiss herdsman of Monroe in his dark blue linen smock rickrack-stitched and a knitted black woolen cap with tassel. Black breeches, white, knitted woolen hose, black garters and black leather shoes.

5. Every five years in Monroe, the American-born descendants of Swiss ancestry don folk costume and celebrate "Cheese Day" with a festival. This young woman is in traditional dress with silver buttons and chains. The apron is of red cotton. The hat is the most traditional piece of the attire, going back centuries and centuries with its horsehair lace loops. The lace is made from the tails and manes of live animals, that being most resilient. In fact, the lace is boiled and baked to retain its kink, then edged with a fabric, here with black velvet, and then sewn to a black velvet hat.

6. An amateur dancer of a Milwaukee troupe which performs for charity, in his heavy white cotton costume, the cape of which is lined with scarlet. The effective decoration consists of black braid, a touch of scarlet embroidery and appliquéd squares of blue faïence. White canvas footwear.

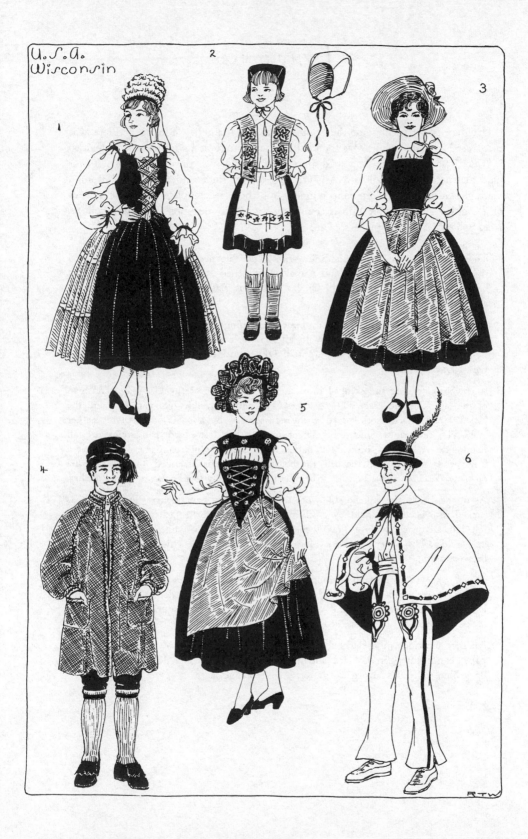

U.S.A.
Wisconsin

❊ *Uruguay* ❊

Plate 106

Uruguay is the smallest of the South American Republics. Rio de la Plata was discovered in 1516, Colona was founded by the Portuguese in 1680 and Montevideo in 1726. The region was long in dispute with the Spanish the final victors. It was held alternately by Brazil and Argentina, becoming independent in 1828. Roman Catholicism is the predominant religion but there is complete tolerance for all other faiths. Primary education is compulsory with all education, including college, free. Spanish is the language spoken.

1. The modern cowhand in white shirt with dark blue neckband, a leather belt and the slim version of the long, full pantaloons fastened at the ankles. Instead of the belt, he sometimes wears a sash. On his head, the Basque berét. Rope-soled canvas alpargatas.

2. A female member of a group of mummers cavorting during the carnival in Montevideo in a dark blue dress sewn with alternating, crinkled paper ruffles of red and white. Her sash and alpargatas are red, white stockings, and a red silk bandana polka-dotted in black.

3. A cowboy attending the carnival in an heirloom costume of the Uruguay plainsman of the late 19th and early 20th centuries. The chiripá, a skirt-like garment, and the jacket are of black cloth edged with red, secured by a silver-ornamented leather belt. The fine white shirt, neckerchief and flaring lace-edged pantaloons are all handmade. A black or brown felt hat is worn over a white bandana. In his belt a knife, and hanging from the belt, the boleadora which is described under Argentina on plate 12. He carries a poncho or blanket and his roomy soft boots are of red leather.

4. As of the 1940's, the gaucho still wore the loose, baggy pantaloons called bombachas tucked into boots and held by a silver-studded leather belt. Jacket, pantaloons and felt hat are black with a gray woolen waistcoat over a white shirt with white neckerchief. His poncho is dark blue striped in gray and white and he carries a broad-strapped riding crop.

5. A youngster of a mummers' group. Shirt and jacket are dark blue decorated with crinkled paper bands of red and yellow. Over the light blue denim bombachas, he has draped an animal skin and on his head, a dark blue Basque berét. Dark blue socks with canvas alpargatas tied with red laces.

6. Another mummer in a dark blue coat made gay with crinkled orange and white paper bands. His shirt is black and his breeches of light blue denim. A straw hat, dark blue socks and alpargatas gartered with orange laces.

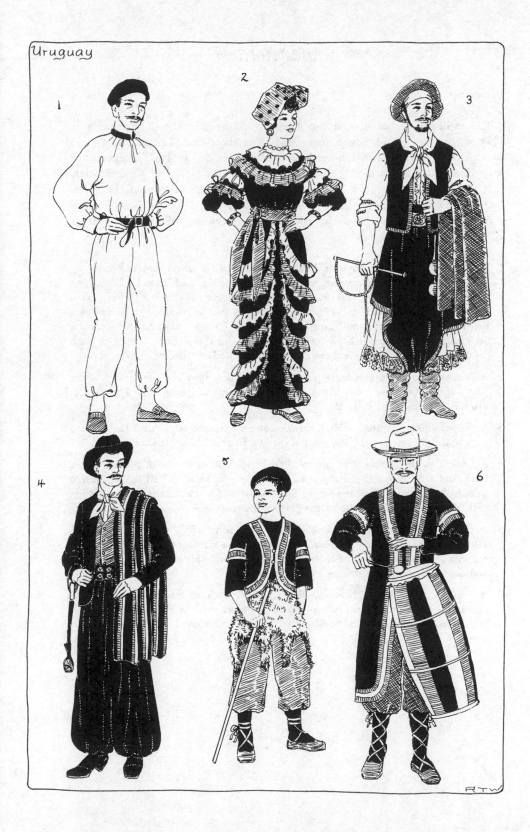

Uruguay

1

2

3

4

5

6

RTW

❧ Venezuela ❧

Plate 107

The earliest historical date of the discovery of the Republic of Venezuela is 1499 when some Spanish navigators coasted along the shores. The first settlement took place by Las Casas in 1520, and Caracas was founded in 1567. Independence was gained from Spain in 1811. From 1819 to 1829 it was part of Colombia but that was terminated in 1850. The present constitution was adopted in 1936. Religious freedom prevails but the religion of the majority is Roman Catholic. Primary education is compulsory with all education, including college, free. Spanish is the language spoken.

1. The torero carrying his capa or "walking cape" of heavy silk made heavier by flower embroidery in colors and conventional motifs in gold thread and colored stones. His dress is a veritable suit of armor reinforced and fitting perfectly as a protection. His exquisitely tucked and frilled white shirt is bound with a sash over which the waistcoat is worn. The slim cravat reaches to the waistline, his stockings are pink or white silk and his slippers are designed for the particular use. The black cap with its ribbon cockade and short pigtail is described on plate 88, number 4.

2. A lovely period gown of salmon pink silk faille worn upon the anniversary of the "days of the Liberator". Self-trimming is in the form of pleats, and a black lace mantilla completes the ensemble.

3. A priest in his street dress, a black cassock buttoned from neck to hem. His hat is a slightly different version of the usual black felt tricorne. Black leather shoes.

4. A Goajira Indian woman with original dress ideas. A flowing robe of printed cotton, black and red on a gold color ground. A frill at the neck and strings of colored wooden beads and a tied bandana for the headdress. The footgear is unique, having dark blue soles with red woolen pompons of fantastic size.

5. A dressy Goajira Indian in a dark blue Western shirt with "snappy" sleevebands. His felt hat, also Western and blue, is banded with a ribbon of matching color. His red and yellow striped loincloth shows below the shirt and on his feet are leather and canvas sandals. He carries a walking stick.

6. A young woman in the traditional festival dress which in these times is fast disappearing. Of salmon pink cotton printed in silver with a dainty white blouse, brightly colored wooden bead necklaces and a pale pink straw hat. Her feet are shod in silver sandals.

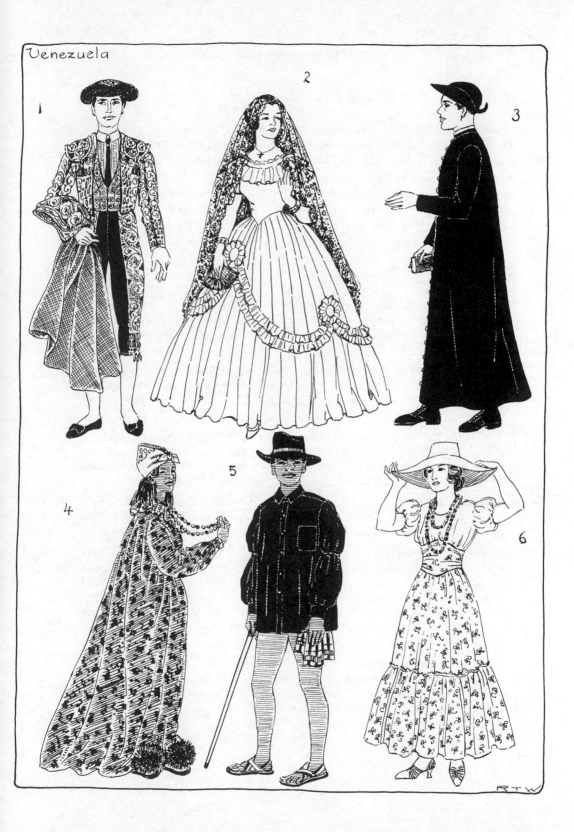

Venezuela

1

2

3

4

5

6

RTW

❊ *Vietnam* ❊

Plate 108

The recorded history of Vietnam, the ancient name of Annam, begins before the Christian Era in Tonkin when settled by the Viets who came from central China. From 11 to 938 A.D. it was ruled by China which was followed by many other periods of vassalage. In 1288 Vietnam defeated Kublai Khan's armies. In the 16th century the French and Portuguese arrived. Cochin China was yielded to France in 1863 and a French protectorate arranged in 1884. In World War II Japan occupied Vietnam which after 1945 was the scene of serious guerrilla warfare between France and the Communists. In 1954, a cease-fire accord divided Vietnam into North and South Vietnam with the promise to settle the country's future, a decision which in this year of 1965 appears explosive.

1. A woman returning from marketing with her purchases in her Oriental wicker carrying-pole. Her costume reveals its Chinese influence in the black skirt called sinhs and the white jacket of cotton or linen. Her straw sun hat is covered with· white cotton on the top side.

2. A Buddhist "Brother of the Saffron Robe" of Hué in his silk robes of saffron and red (red designated by black in our illustration) worn over white cotton trousers. Saffron silk cap, white socks and gray sandals, and in his hands, the black tasseled and colored stones prayer chain.

3. The contemporary version of the traditional costume of the Annam or Vietnamese women. A semi-fitted chemise or oudai, here in a sheer silk of sky-blue printed with a rose and white floral design. Underneath, black silk or velvet pantaloons and on her head, the large sun straw hat and on her feet, black banded sandals.

4. A priest making his morning rounds for rice furnished by Buddhist followers. He carries a bowl with a saffron-colored cover. The draped robe, which is a straight piece of fabric, is saffron-colored because this is supposedly the most peaceful of colors.

5. A young mother carrying her baby in a sling fastened to her body by heavy tapes crossed over the chest and tied in front. Her dress is black silk and the wrap-around leggings black cloth. Mother and baby wear ivory bracelets and baby, a blue and white checked jumper and an orange berét. Among the Vietnamese there are three sets according to the districts in which they live, Black Thais who wear black blouses, White Thais who wear white blouses and Red Thais who wear red blouses, but are not Communists.

6. A prince of Hué in a beautifully embroidered tunic or cai-co of plum-colored satin. The flowers are white and turquoise blue with a touch of red and the Chinese motif in gold color. His trousers or caiquan are white linen over white socks and black patent leather slippers. The smart cap is dull black silk with the headband laid in tiny folds (see sketch below).

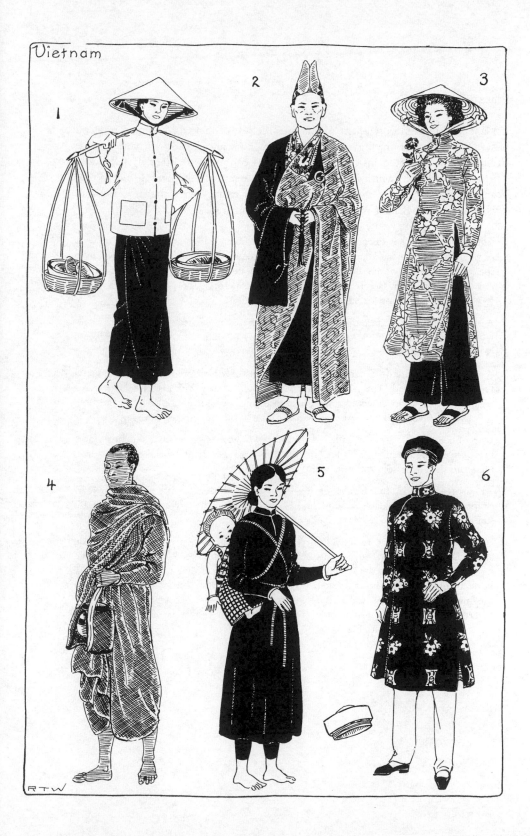

Vietnam

1   2   3

4   5   6

RTW

✻ *Yemen* ✻

Plate 109

Yemen, a kingdom in southern Arabia, was the seat of the old Minaean Kingdom. It was conquered by the Egyptians about 1600 B.C. and invaded in turn by the Ethiopians and the Romans. In 628 A.D. it was converted to Islam. It fell under Turkish control from which it acquired a large measure of autonomy before World War I. In 1934, after intermittent border warfare, treaties were made with Saudi Arabia and Great Britain regulating Yemen's boundaries.

1. The use of the veil is disappearing among Arab women but this woman is a resident of Sa'na, the capital of Yemen, where it is still required in public. Over the chalwar she wears a heavy woven shawl, the center done in French blue and the border in red and yellow. Her face is covered by the yashmak or black purdah veil and her feet are dressed in canvas slippers and red stockings.

2. A crown prince in a beautiful Moslem robe, the aba, of heavy plum-colored silk with lapels of a deeper hue and batik-dyed motifs in dull red. A wide embroidered belt holds his knife and amber prayer-beads.

3. A native of Hodeida in a flaring bolero the sleeves of which are skin-tight and therefore must be knitted. The jacket is tan with brown stripes. His nether garment, the serul, is a long strip of white cotton, wrapped and tied forming short breeches and a pocket to hold his knife. Also of white cotton is his self-draped turban.

4. One of a group of women gathered at the town well, all dressed alike in a large black shawl bordered with white crochet lace. A sash holds the shawl in place. Underneath can be seen the slim white cotton chalwar.

5. An army officer in full regalia of black turban and jacket with a sky-blue scarf draped over his shoulders. Around his waist, a waterproofed white poncho and his knife in the belt.

6. A young prince dressed to attend a reception. A black turban and a yellow cotton aba striped in black. A fringed scarf striped red, black and yellow is wrapped round his body and he carries the jambiya in his belt. Every man or boy carries the curved knife in his belt when he is dressed. Dagger handles are of wood or horn, the latter the most expensive. The scabbard is covered with dyed leather tape or ribbon, the favorite color seemingly bright blue. The powder horn shown is of horn and gold work with chain of gold beads.

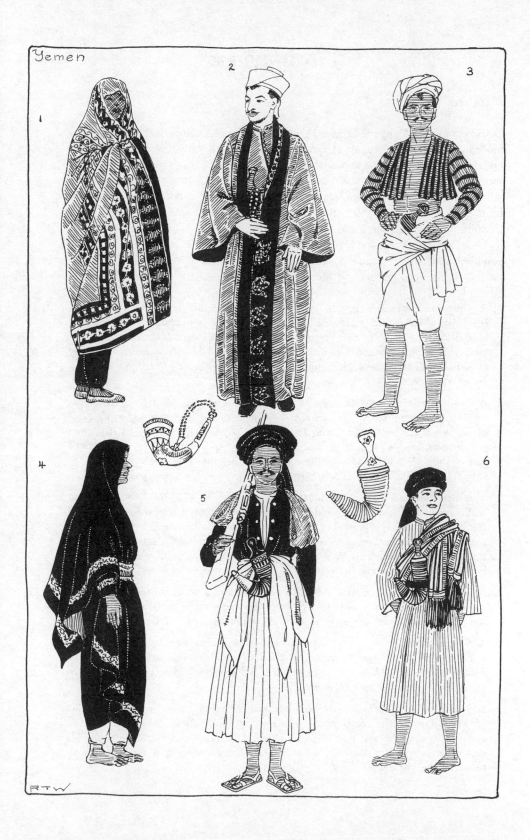

Yemen

❧ *Yugoslavia* ❧

Plate 110

Six republics make up the Federal Peoples' Republic of Yugoslavia: Serbia, Croatia, Slovenia, Montenegro, Bosnia-Herzogovina and Macedonia. When the Austrian archduke and his wife were assassinated at Sarajevo in 1914, the Austrian government went to war against Serbia and brought on World War I. Upon the collapse of the Austro-Hungarian Empire, a kingdom was formed of the states. This was invaded by the Germans in 1941. A national liberation movement under Marshal Tito, a Communist, defeated the invaders and proclaimed Yugoslavia a Federal Republic in 1945. Elementary training is compulsory but all education is free. All religions are equal in rights with forty-two percent following the Serbian Orthodox faith, Roman Catholics thirty-two percent and Moslems twelve percent.

1. A prosperous Dalmatian peasant wearing his centuries-old, family heirloom dress. It consists of bolero and jacket with slashed hanging sleeves in black, or perhaps dark blue cloth embroidered in gold or gold colored thread. A sword is thrust through the wide red woolen sash and a red kerchief is tied round his head. The trousers are fashioned in Turkish style, the white blouse is of hand-loomed linen and the shoes are of rawhide.

2. A Croatian matron in white linen blouse and white woolen skirt, both homespun, the blouse embroidered in brilliant red and yellow. The collarless jacket of black or red felt is also embroidered and appliquéd in gay colors. The fringed felt apron is colorfully hand-worked in a design different for each village. The long knitted socks, white for maids and dark blue for matrons, repeat the bright colors of the costume. A white headcloth floats from the tiny kapa in black and red.

3. The men's national costume of Montenegro. A tunic of white or light blue cloth with sash of red, brown and gold silk is worn over a double-breasted vest of red silk bordered with gold braid. Over the tunic, a red cloth bolero with hanging sleeves braided or embroidered in gold color, and under the vest the white linen shirt. The knee breeches are dark blue cloth in Turkish style, with white gaiters and rawhide shoes completing the costume.

4. A Serb in all-white linen with a full-skirted tunic over a white shirt and pantaloons cut in Turkish style. His wide sash makes a fine carry-all for small necessaries. The smart cap is black astrakan and the shoes are white canvas in Western fashion.

5. A Serbian girl spinning yarn from wool and wearing her own handiwork of roses and lilacs stitched in needlepoint. A black cloth corselet over a white linen blouse and an embroidered black felt apron over her red and black plaid woolen skirt. The young lady wears her hair in two braids.

6. A young man of Bosnia in dark blue buckskin or velvet bolero and knee breeches of Turkish style. The colors of the silk sash are red, yellow and black, and red and yellow edge the vest with the embroidery in dark red. A white linen shirt, a dark blue cap with red crown, white woolen knitted socks and rawhide sandals make up the picturesque dress.

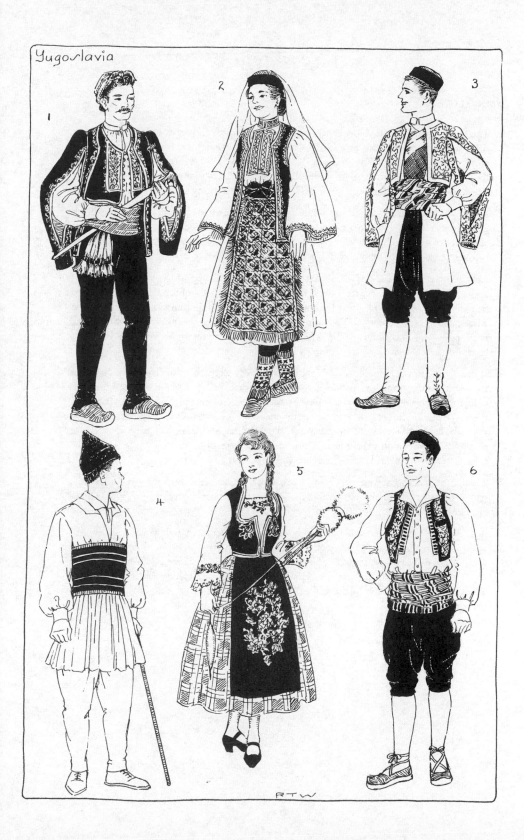

Yugoslavia

RTW

❧ *Yugoslavia* ❧

Plate III

1. The rich dress of this Slovene farmer's daughter is composed of three different silks. Cap and corselet are brocaded in a yellow rose motif on a maroon ground and edged with a narrow velvet ribbon. The skirt is dark blue brocaded in black but the plum-colored apron is of brocade all in one tone. Of white lawn are the bonnet ties and the blouse. Slippers are black with white stockings.

2. A gay Macedonian costume in white homespun linen with red, gray and black embroidery. The bolero and cap are black, the latter sparked with a falcon feather and red crown. The breeches follow the Turkish pattern with wonderful hand-knitted woolen socks of red, yellow and black and rawhide sandals.

3. The Sunday dress of a girl of Slovak ancestry. A full cotton skirt, white with pink, and a white linen blouse with ribbon beading. The starched, embroidered triple-ruffled sleeves have bowknots of deep pink ribbon. And most important is the black apron with brilliant embroidery. The young woman wears two headkerchiefs, one black with pink and the outer one, white with pink. Very smart indeed are her soft, black leather boots.

4. A Serbian Orthodox monk wearing the dalmatic and tiara. The complete habit in its beauty and simplicity symbolizes artistic purity and perfection of design. The dalmatic originated in Dalmatia where it was noted and copied by Roman visitors in the days of the emperors. Also worn by the early Christians, it became ecclesiastic vestment and royal raiment in the West. The Dalmatian sleeve has been in and out of the Western mode ever since. Tiara and robe are of fine, dull black cloth, the robe fastened to one side with tasseled cords.

5. Though the Bosnian woman discards the feredeza at home or in the country, she still adheres strictly to the old customs when on city streets by wearing a light-colored or checked dorino and a black yashmak.

6. A Dalmatian miss in a dark blue cloth tunic embroidered in red, yellow, green and white. The Dalmatian-sleeved blouse, vest and skirt are of white linen with vest and blouse embroidered in blue and white. The skirt is fashioned in four wide box pleats and the sash is dark blue silk. Her headgear is formed of two scarfs, one fringed and striped and the other plain white. Rawhide sandals and varicolored knitted socks dress her feet.

Yugoslavia

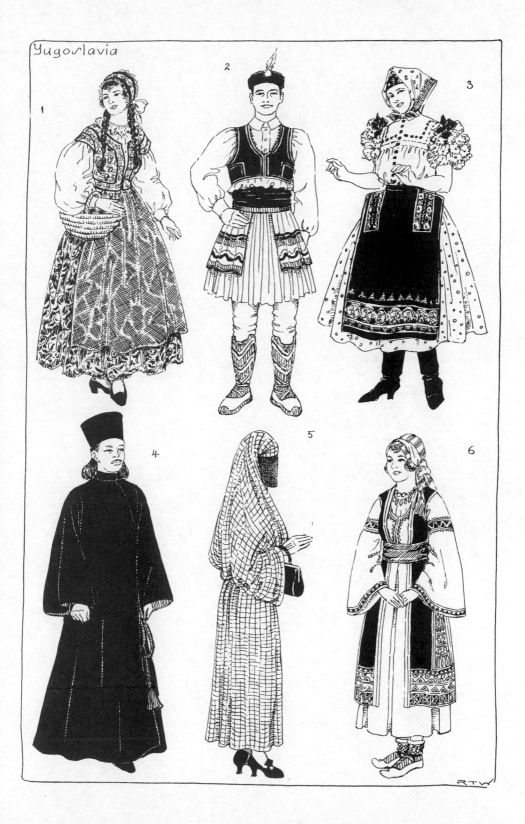

RTW

❧ *Bibliography* ❧

A Dictionary of Men's Wear—William Harry Baker—Cleveland, 1908

Album of American History—James Truslow Adams—Charles Scribner's Sons —New York, 1944

A Pageant of Hats, Ancient and Modern—Ruth Edwards Kilgour—New York, 1958

A Picture History of Russia—John Stuart Marten—Crown Publishers, New York, 1945

Ciba Review—Indian Costume #36—Swiss Peasant #55—Basle, Switzerland

Costume Throughout the Ages—Mary Evans—J. B. Lippincott Company, Philadelphia, 1930

Designs, Forms and Ornaments—Michael Estrui—Knickerbocker Publishing Company, New York, 1947

Dictionaire du Costume—Maurice Leloir—Paris, 1951

Die Trachten der Volker—Albert Kretschmer—Leipsic, 1906

Early American Costume—Warwick and Pitz—New York, 1929

Encyclopaedia Britannica—11th Edition, New York, 1911

Encyclopedia of Costume—James Robinson Planché—London, 1876

Encyclopedia, Funk and Wagnall's New Standard—New York and London, 1937

Encyclopedia of Textiles—Renate Jaques and Ernest Flemming—Frederick A. Praeger Inc., New York, 1958

Historic Costume for the Stage—Lucy Barton—New York, 1938

Indians of America—Lillian Davids Fazzino—Wisconsin, 1935

Indians—American Heritage—New York, 1961

Indians of the Americas—National Geographic Society—Washington, D.C., 1955

Le Costume Historique—M. A. Racinet—Firmin Didot et Cie., Paris, 1888

Les Costumes—Anciens et Modernes—Fr. Hottenroth—E. Weyhe, New York

Münchner Bilderbogen, Zur Geschichte der Kostüme—Braun & Schneider—Munich, late 19th century

National Geographic Magazine—Washington, D.C.—1908 to 1964

Peasant Costume in Europe—Kathleen Mann—Macmillan Company, New York —1950

Textile Folk Art—Antonin Vaclavik & Jaroslav Orel—Spring Books, London

The American Indian—Oliver La Farge—Crown Publishers Inc., New York—1956

The Book of Costume by a Lady of Rank—London 1847

The Book of Indians—Holling and Holling—New York, 1935

The Bulletins of the Metropolitan Museum of Art—New York

The Grammar of Ornament—Owen Jones—Leonard Quaritch, London—1910

The History of American Costume—Elizabeth McClellan, George W. Jacobs & Co., New York—1910 and 1942

The Illustrated Library of the World and Its Peoples—Greystone Press—New York, 1964

The Language of Fashion—Mary Brooks Picken—New York, 1939

The Life World Library—Time Inc.—New York, 1964

The Look of the Old West—Foster-Harris—New York, 1955

The Regional Costumes of Spain—Isabel de Palencia—Spain, 1926

The Slovak National Dress Through the Centuries—Josef Markov—Artia, Prague, 1956

Trachten Unserer Zeit—Heinz Hecker—Callweg, Munich—1939

Webster's Geographical Dictionary—publishers G. and C. Merriam Company—Springfield, Mass., 1949

Webster's New International Dictionary—2nd Edition—G. and C. Merriam Company, Springfield, Mass., 1937

100,000 Years of Daily Life—Jacques Broisse, Paul Chaland, Jacques Ostier—Golden Press—New York, 1961

✳ Index ✳